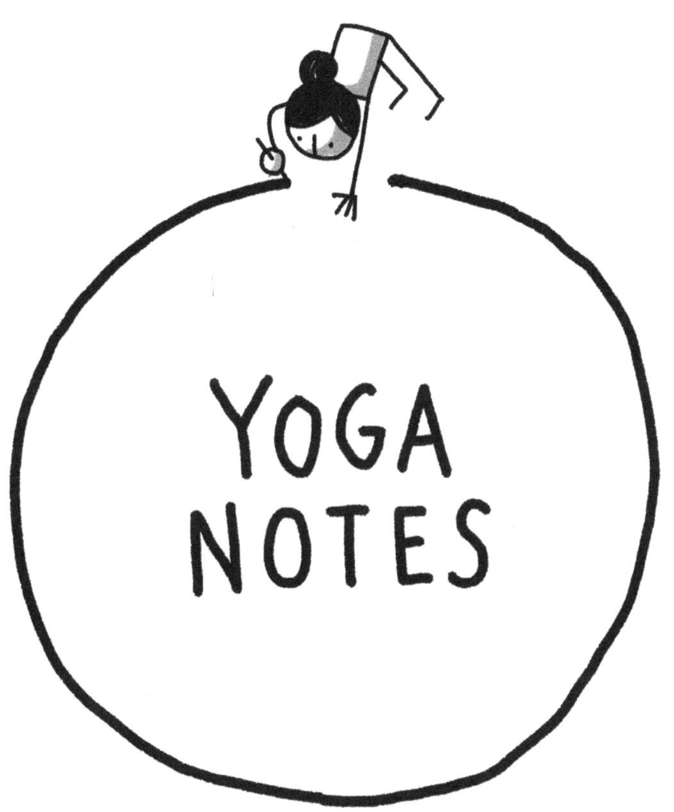

YOGA NOTES

How to SKETCH
YOGA POSTURES
& SEQUENCES

A GUIDE by EVA-LOTTA LAMM

ISBN 978-3-9820693-0-2

Self-published
by Eva-Lotta Lamm, Berlin

First published in 2018
2nd Edition, January 2019

www.yoganotes.net

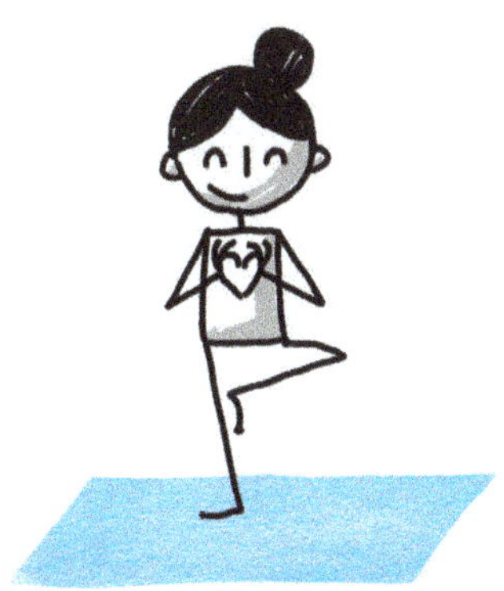

DISCLAIMER

This book is not meant to teach you the yoga postures shown. I strongly recommend that you study yoga with a good teacher who will show you how to practice each posture safely, who will point out the modifications that are right for your body and your level and who will correct your alignment during practice.

Learning face-to-face from an experienced teacher is the best way to build a safe, confident and enjoyable yoga practice.

WHAT THIS BOOK CONTAINS

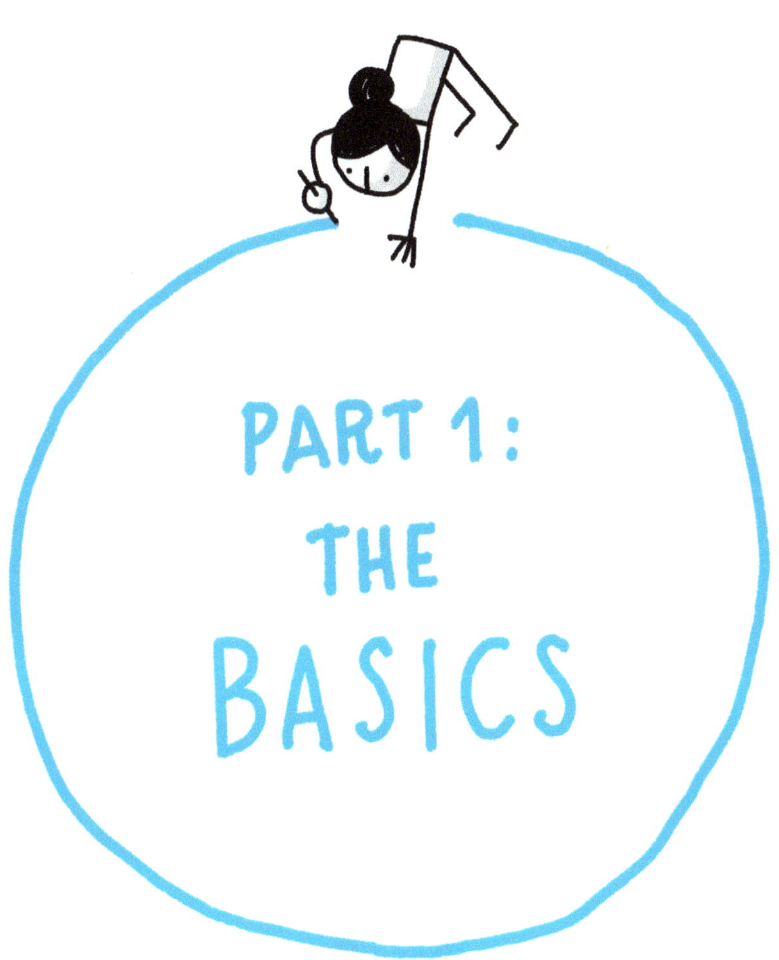

PART 1:
THE
BASICS

WHO IS THIS BOOK FOR?

This book is for anybody who is studying, practicing or teaching yoga and who wants to be able to take simple visual notes for their practice, classes or training course.

Sketching is a quick and simple way to capture information, to remember it better and to communicate with other people. Capturing and expressing information visually supports learning and understanding. Visuals are a great complement to practical learning and verbal explanations.

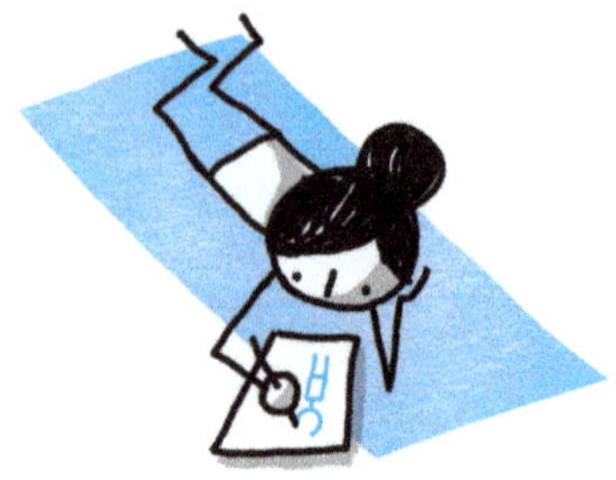

Sketching yoga sequences can be helpful for yoga practitioners and teachers who want to deepen their understanding or share their knowledge with others.

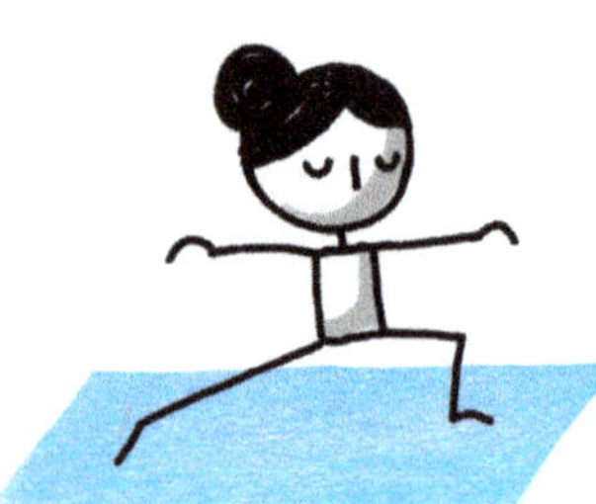

STUDENTS & PRACTITIONERS

If you study or practice yoga, you can sketch out your favourite sequences to use as a guide during your home practice or for when you are travelling. Sketch out that great class you attended at your yoga studio or the nice flow you found on YouTube. The sketched overview will be the perfect cheat sheet to keep by your mat during your own practice.

TEACHER TRAINING ATTENDEES

If you are learning to be a yoga teacher there is a lot of information to take in and to process. Taking visual notes and using sketches to capture the details about postures, alignment and anatomy will help you to get the most out of your training. The notes you create will be clearer, more engaging and actually fun to look at and revise again later.

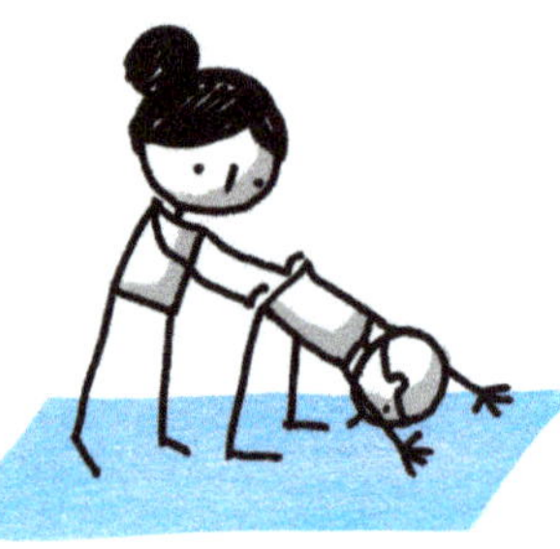

YOGA TEACHERS & COACHES

If you teach yoga classes or work with private clients, sketch to plan sequences and create practice plans in a visual way. You can use them as a visual overview during class (if you haven't fully memorised the sequence yet). They also make great handouts for your students after a workshop or as personalised practice plans for your one-on-one clients.

"... BUT I CAN'T DRAW!"

You might think of yourself as somebody who "can't draw" or who has no talent for art. Don't worry. Sketching is not about creating art, but about capturing information and expressing ideas. We are not trying to create realistic life drawings, but to sketch simple, but clear little icons that help us to remember a sequence of postures.

Learning to sketch is a bit like learning to write. It takes a bit of effort in the beginning and some continued practice, but after some time, it will feel like second nature.

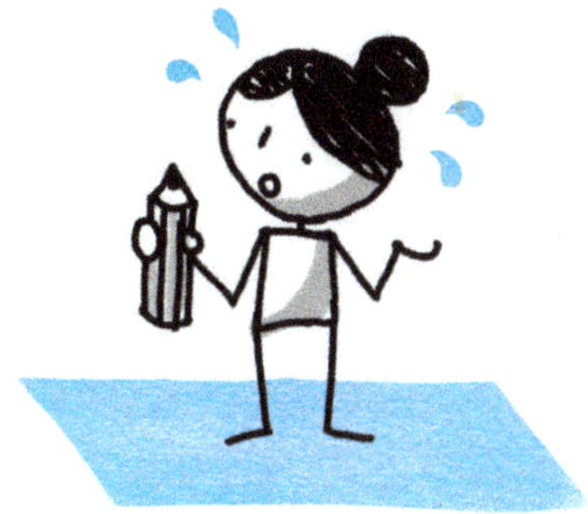

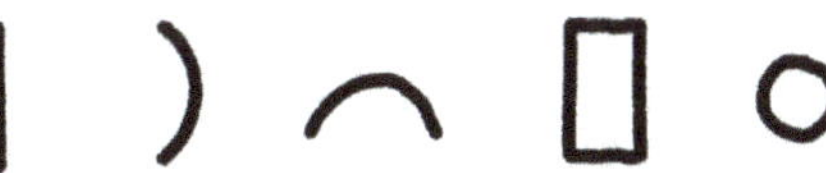

All we need to start is less than a handful of simple shapes: Straight lines, curved lines, rectangles and circles. We then put these together in different ways to sketch any kind of asana. It's a bit like Lego.

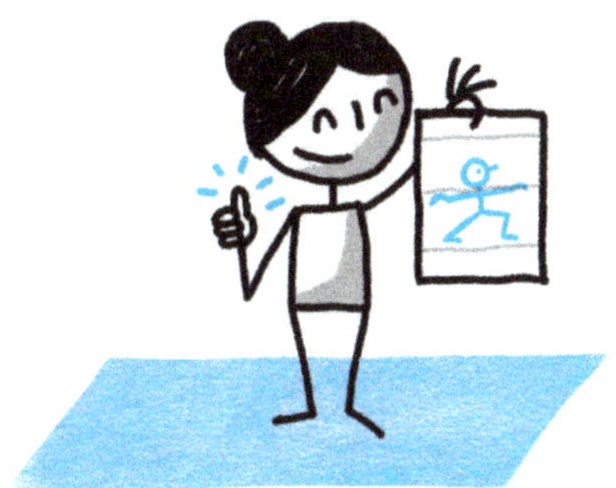

In the first part of the book, we will learn the basic principles of how to build up an asana sketch. I also share some handy tricks throughout the book that will help you to get a pro at sketching yoga notes in no time.

The second part of the book shows you how to sketch more than 80 asanas step by step along with variations, preparation and related poses. This will help you to practice each asana specifically using the principles you learned in part 1.

PRACTICE, AND ALL IS COMING

Like yoga, sketching is a practice. It is not about creating a perfect beautiful pose, but about the experience and insight we gain when we practice. Don't worry about your sketches being ugly or not good enough.

As long as your sketches help you to remember a flow or to capture some alignment detail you don't want to forget, they do their job. They are good enough. And they will get better with every asana you sketch.

Oh, and don't forget to keep breathing while you sketch ;)

PERSPECTIVE

We are trying to simplify our sketches as
much as possible. This includes simplifying
the perspective. For each asana, we chose
one of three views that shows the most
information about the posture.

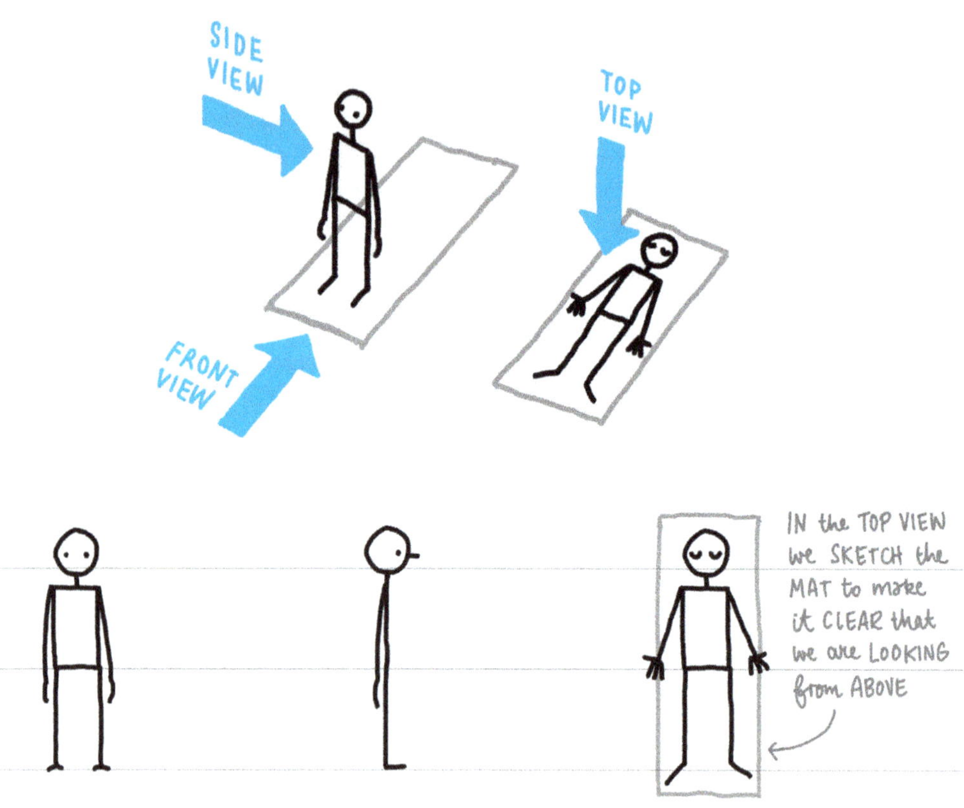

FRONT VIEW

In the front view, we sketch
the torso as a rectangle. This
gives us a clear view of both
shoulders and hips where the
arms and legs attach.

SIDE VIEW

In the side view, we reduce
the torso to a single line.
When both arms or both legs
are in the same position, we
sketch them as one.

TOP VIEW

In the top view, we look at
the body from above as if we
were hovering over the mat.
To distinguish a top view from
a front / side view, we sketch
the mat underneath the body.

There are a few asanas where neither of the
three simple views gives us a clear picture of
the posture. In these cases, we can mix two
views – front and top view or side and top
view – to show the most information possible.

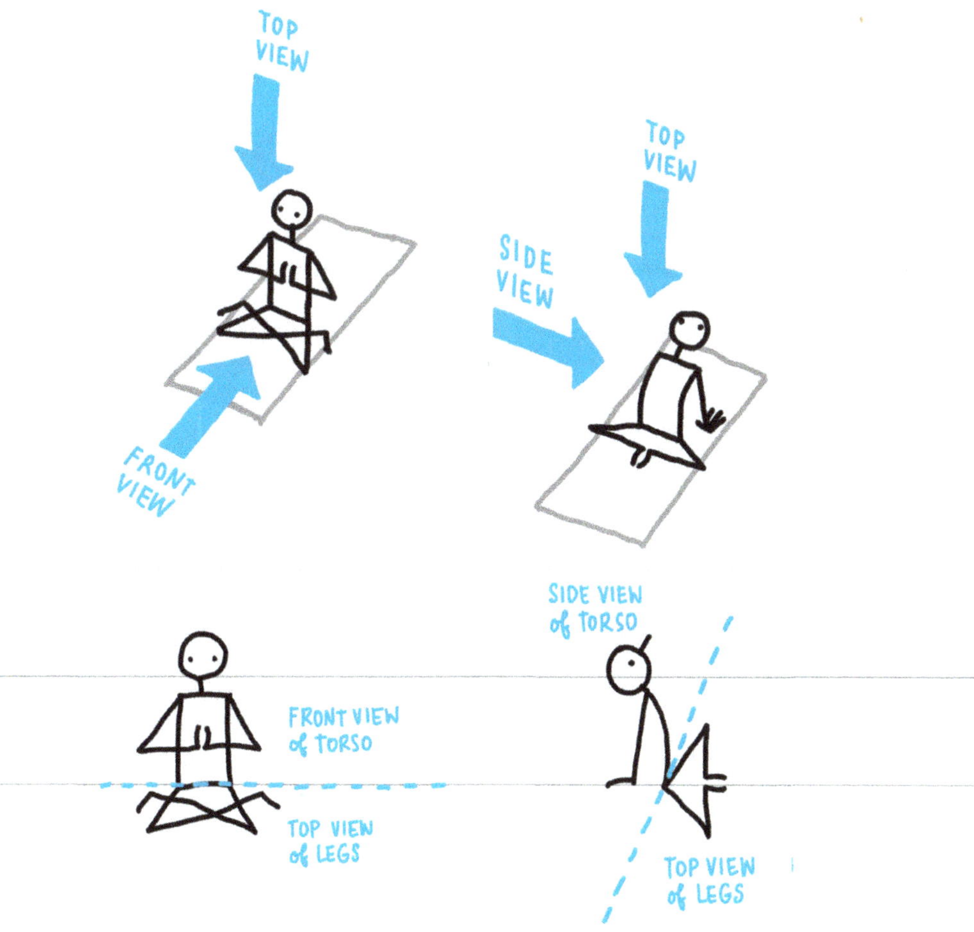

Remember, we are not trying to do a life
drawing but to think of our sketch as a
schematic or diagram. If mixing perspectives
adds clarity, this kind of "cheating" is allowed.

USING THE BASE LINE

The baseline represents the floor. Anchoring our sketches on the ground helps us to follow a sequence and see at a glance when it transitions from standing to sitting to lying.

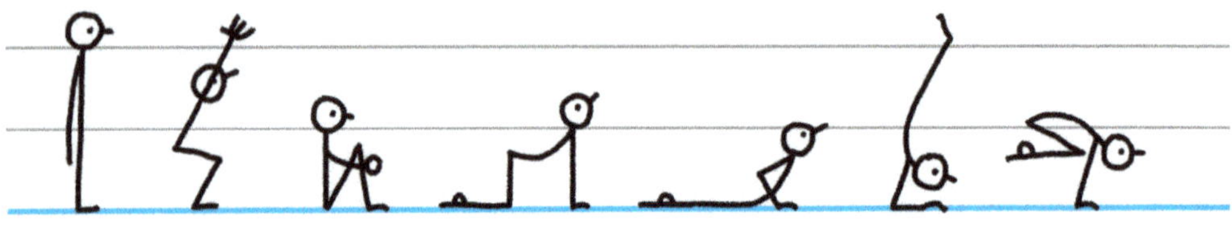

In standing postures the feet are grounded on the baseline. If the feet rotate, the heel is the part that stays on the base line.

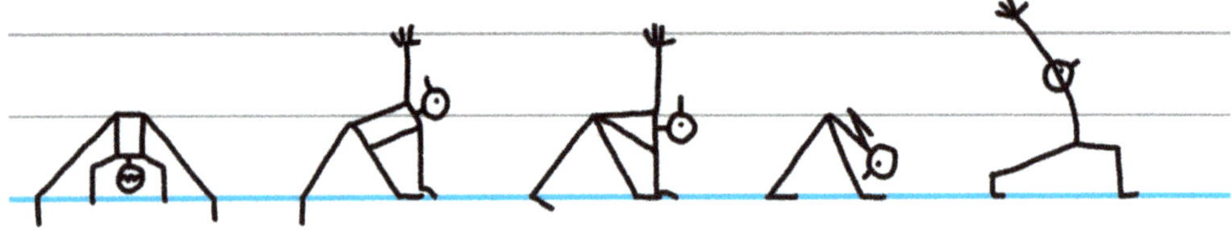

In sitting positions the buttocks are grounded on the baseline. The torso rises up from there and any parts extending towards the viewer extend below the baseline.

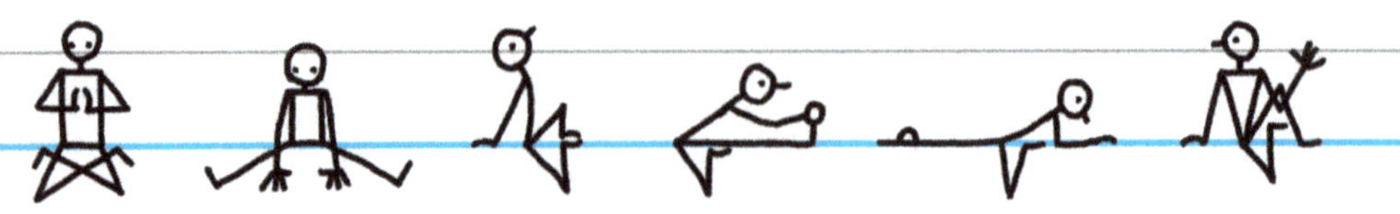

PROPORTIONS

An average adult is about 7 heads tall. To simplify the proportions for sketching, we go roughly with the following measurements:

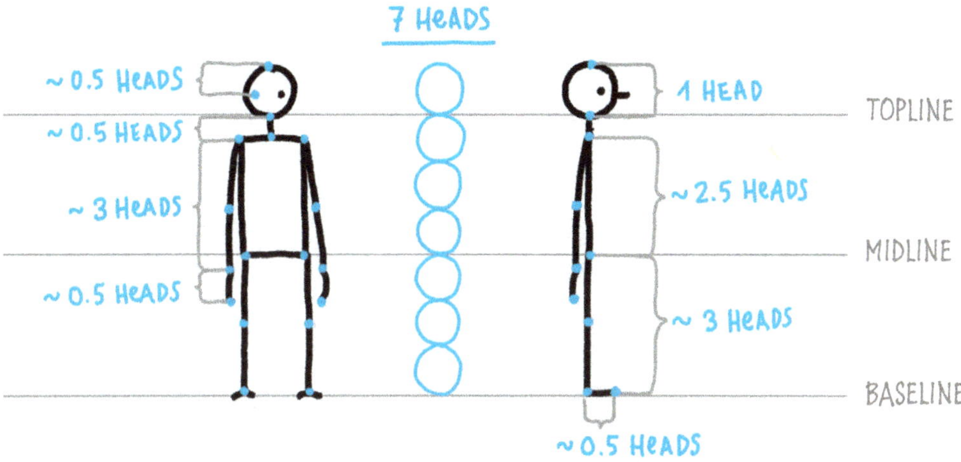

Legs: ~ 3 heads
Legs go from baseline to midline, knees in the middle.

Feet: ~ 0.5 heads

Torso: ~ 2.5 heads

Neck: ~ 0.5 heads
Torso and neck fit into the space from midline to topline line.

Arms: ~ 2.5–3 heads
A little bit longer than the torso, from shoulders to just below the hips.

Hands: ~ 0.5 heads
When arms and hands are hanging alongside the body, the fingertips are reaching to the middle of the thighs.

Head: 1 head ;)
Nose and eyes are halfway down the head.

GETTING PROPORTIONS RIGHT

Getting the proportion of your sketches right can be a bit tricky at first, but with some practice you will get a natural feel for the right length of each part.

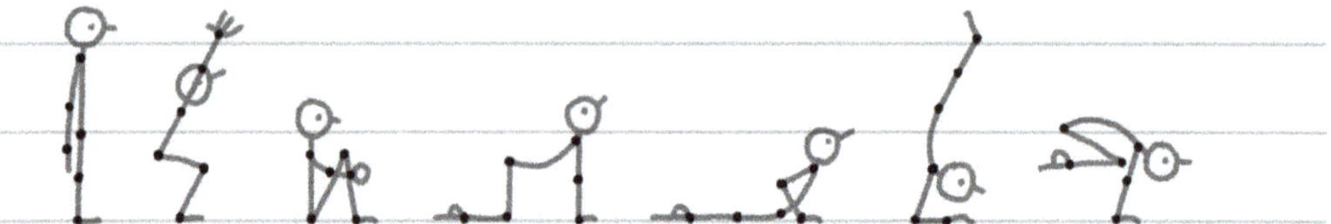

In the beginning you can try to add dots at the knees and elbows – especially on straight legs and arms. This gives a bit more structure and helps with measuring the length of extended limbs.

Remember, it is not about being 100% anatomically correct, but about getting the lengths of the body parts right enough to represent the essence of the asana. If an arm ends up a bit too long, a leg too short, or the head a bit too big, it's not the end of the world.

SKETCHING STEP-BY-STEP

The order in which we sketch the poses can help with getting the proportions and positioning of the different body parts right.

GROUNDING FIRST

I like to start by anchoring the body in the space. For most postures this means "grounding" the body by sketching the part that is touching the floor first. This gives me a good basis and handy reference points for building up the rest of the pose.

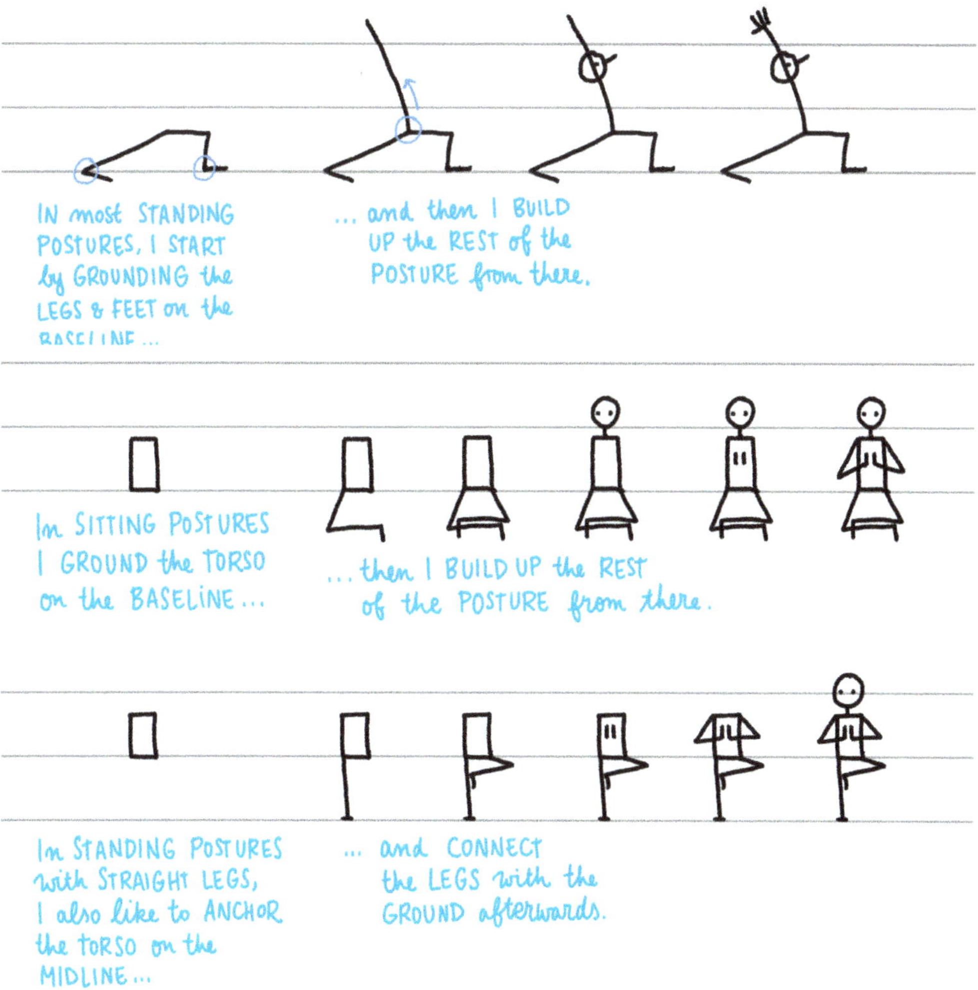

FINDING THE RIGHT SIZE

We all have our own comfort size when it comes to sketching. When I ask you to sketch a square, a circle and a triangle on an empty piece of paper, they will probably end up at roughly the same size every time you do this exercise. This is your comfort zone. Usually, the less confident people are in their sketching abilities, the smaller they tend to sketch.

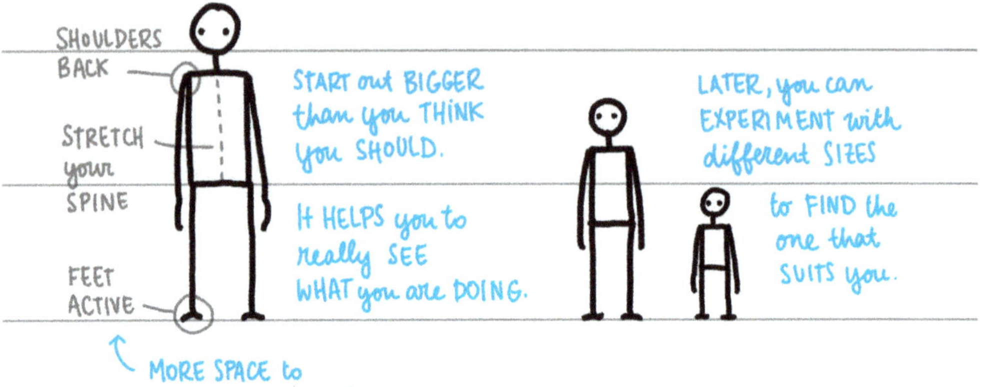

I encourage you to make your sketches bigger, at least in the beginning. Sketching bigger might feel uncomfortable at first, but it makes it much easier for you to see what is going on. Sketching bigger also leaves room to add annotations about alignment or movement.

Try sketching in different sizes and see what suits you and the occasion. If you are focussing on alignment and want to add lots of notes, go bigger. If you are just creating a little cheat sheet of a flow you are already relatively familiar with, you can go very small.

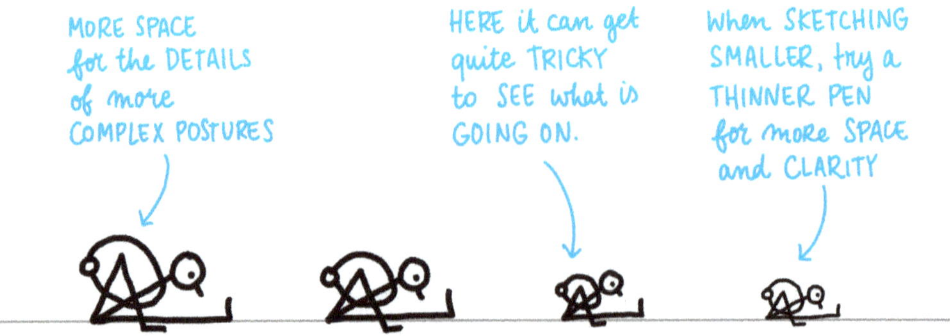

LEVEL OF DETAIL

In this book, I am showing all the postures with full detail. I sketch out the position of the hands, feet and the head (by adding a nose pointing in the direction of the gaze).
We can also sketch a simplified version without these details.

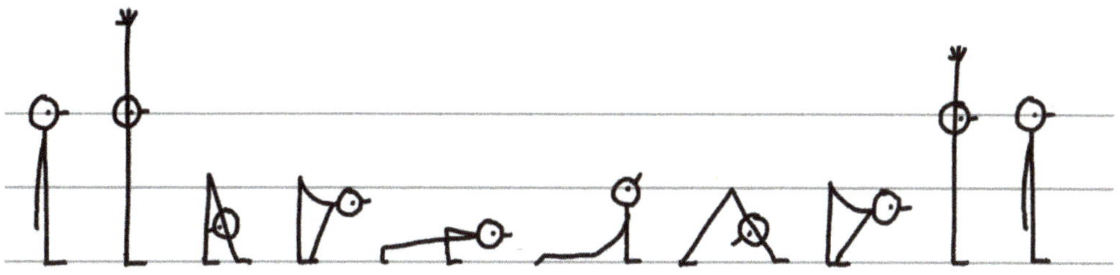

DETAILED

Sketching this "shorthand" version is quicker and good enough to remember a sequence of poses we are already quite familiar with.

It's also possible to mix levels of detail within the same sequence,

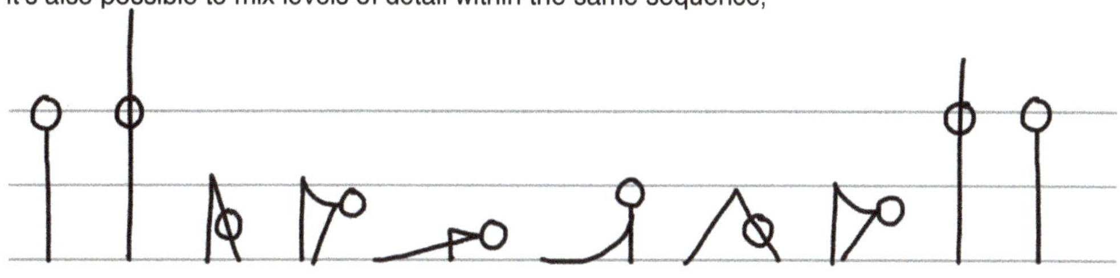

SIMPLIFIED

and even within the same asana sketch. If we are sketching a familiar posture with a new variation (for example the hand position), we sketch a simplified version of the posture and then just add detail for the part that is new. Mixing the level of detail in this way shifts the visual focus onto the detailed part, which is great to highlight new or different elements.

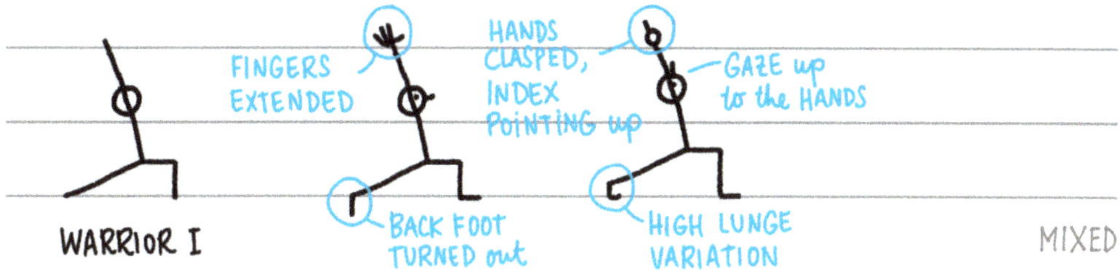

CLARITY OVER REALISM

We already learned in the sections on perspective and proportion that we are trying to maximise the clarity of our sketches and that we are happy to sacrifice realism in some areas in return for a clearer sketch.

Here are a few more small tricks we can apply to enhance the clarity in areas that get visually dense and complex, especially when body parts touch, overlap or cross.

TOUCHING BODY PARTS

When two body parts touch it can be hard to distinguish a touch from a crossing and to keep track of which body part is which before and after the touch. To reduce confusion we can leave just a little gap between the two touching parts. We sketch them really close but we don't make the lines touch.

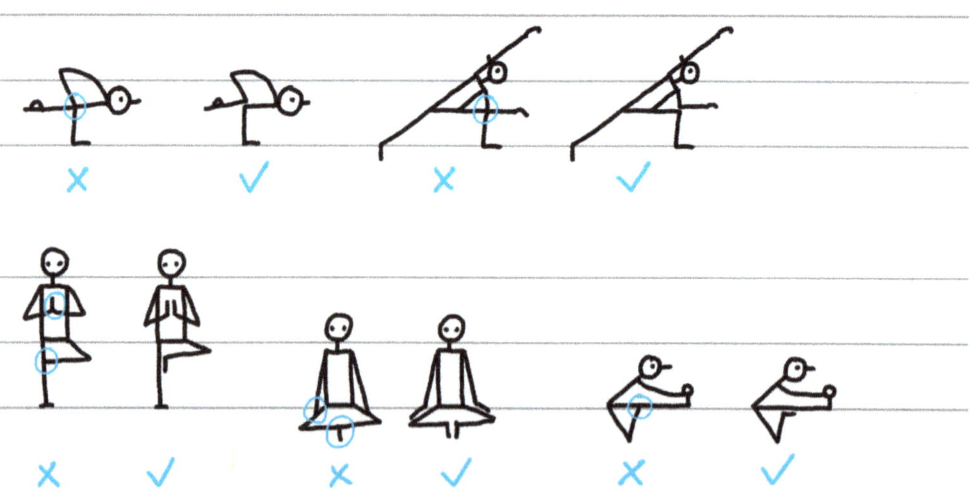

OVERLAPPING BODY PARTS

When two body parts run alongside or in
front of each other, like the arm hanging
alongside the torso in a side view, we sketch
them as slightly separated, parallel lines.

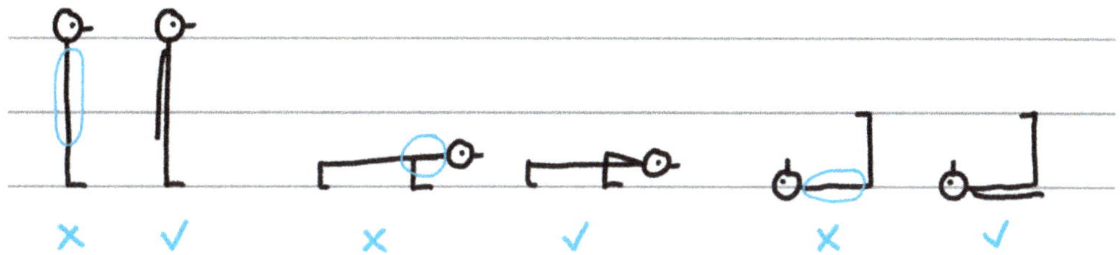

CROSSING BODY PARTS

Similar to touching, a crossing of two limbs
can be visually confusing, especially when
the crossing happens exactly in the joints.
To reach more visual clarity, we don't sketch
the crossing directly in the joint. Instead, we
let the limbs cross a little before or after.

If there are multiple crossings (like in eagle
pose) or the limbs cross really tightly (like in
some binds) we leave some extra space in
our sketch to make it easier for the eyes to
follow the different lines and to understand
what is going on.

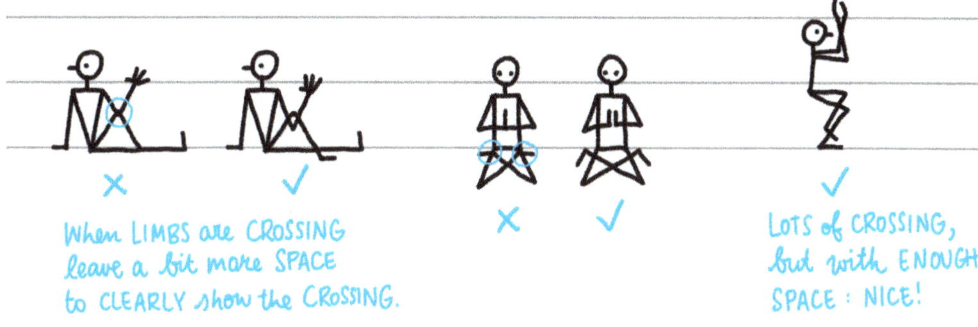

INDIVIDUAL BODY PARTS AND THEIR BASIC VARIATIONS

In this section we will go through the individual body parts and have a closer look at some standard positions and how to sketch them. This basic vocabulary of parts will help us to sketch the different asanas in part 2. We can combine the basics to sketch more variations and modifications that go beyond the postures shown in this book.

LEGS AND FEET
STANDING LEG AND FEET VARIATIONS

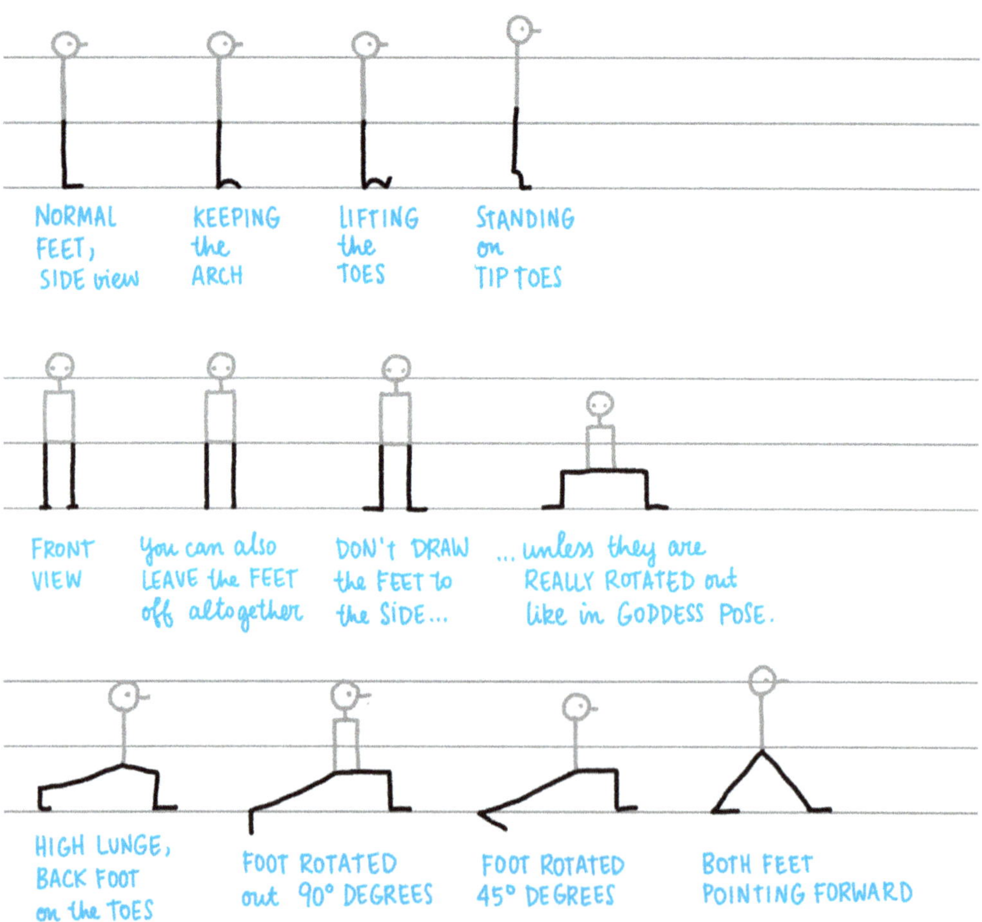

KNEELING AND SITTING LEG AND FEET VARIATIONS

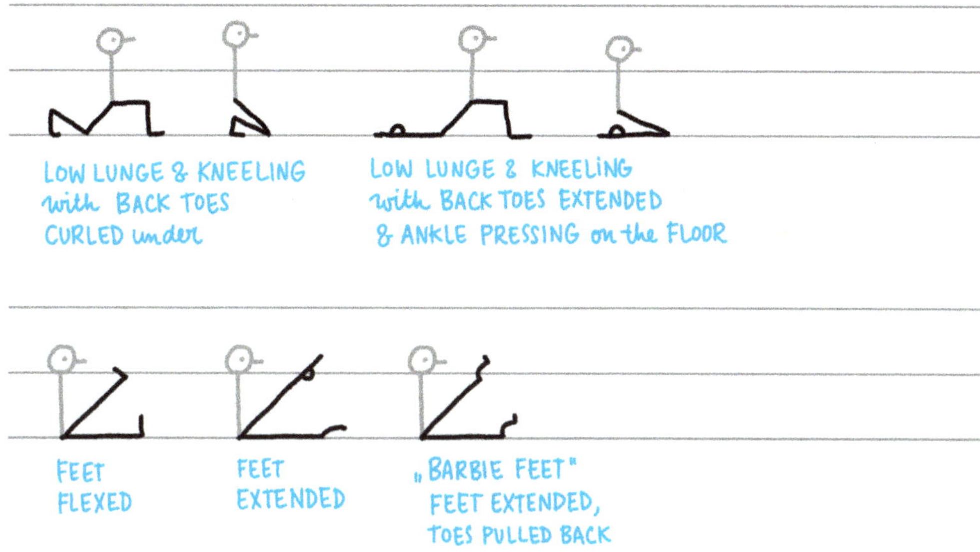

LOW LUNGE & KNEELING
with BACK TOES
CURLED under

LOW LUNGE & KNEELING
with BACK TOES EXTENDED
& ANKLE PRESSING on the FLOOR

FEET
FLEXED

FEET
EXTENDED

„BARBIE FEET"
FEET EXTENDED,
TOES PULLED BACK

SOME MORE CLASSIC LEG VARIATIONS

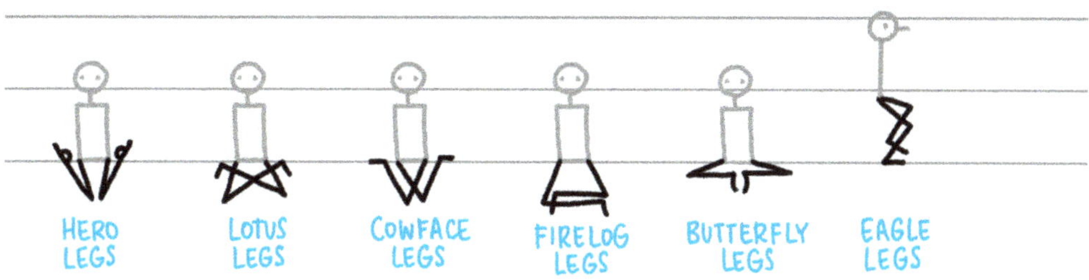

HERO
LEGS

LOTUS
LEGS

COWFACE
LEGS

FIRELOG
LEGS

BUTTERFLY
LEGS

EAGLE
LEGS

ARMS AND HANDS

BASIC ARM AND HAND POSITIONS

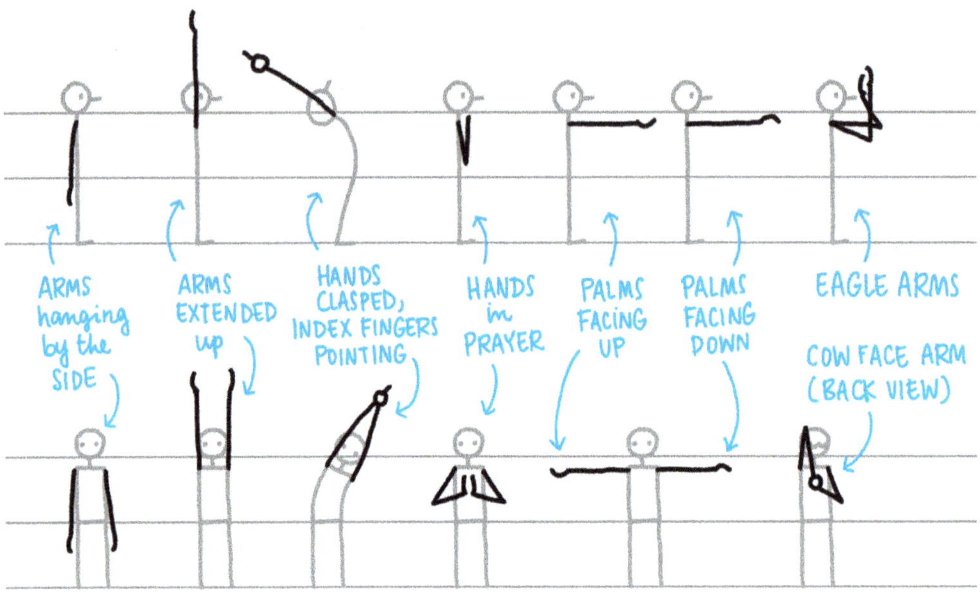

HOLDING AND BINDING

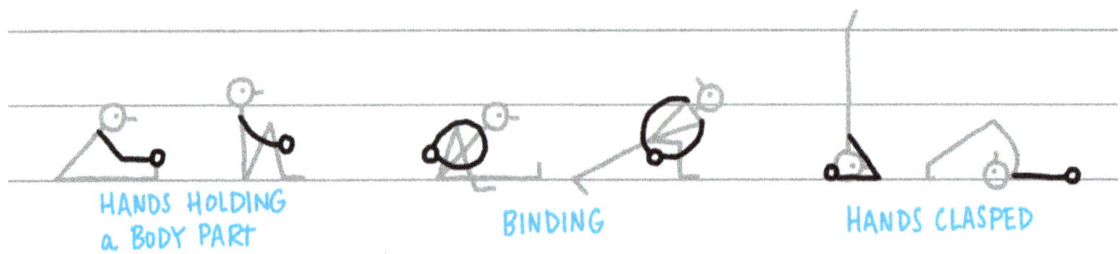

EXTENDED FINGERS

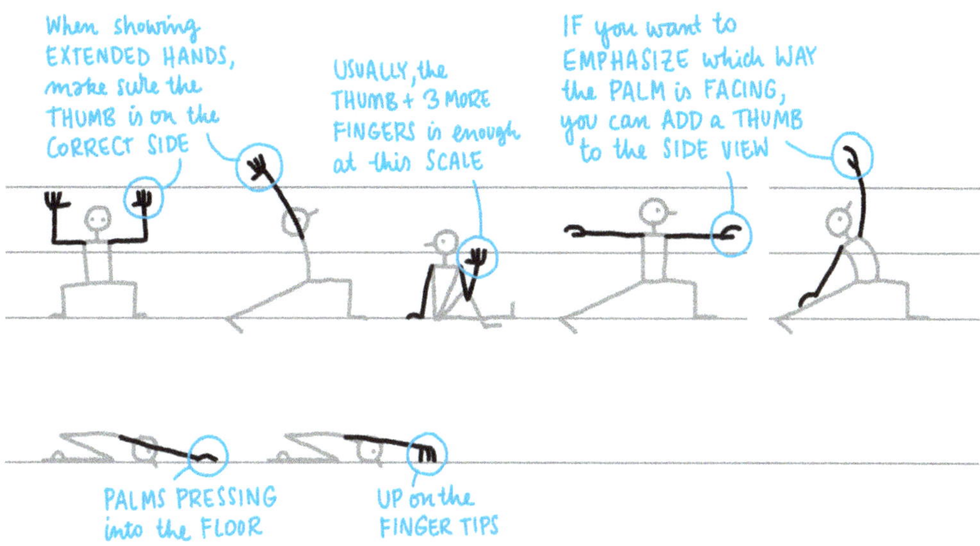

MUDRAS

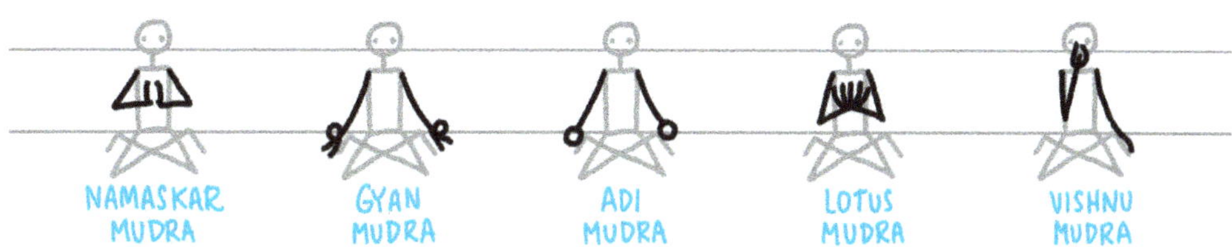

TORSO

BASIC POSITIONS

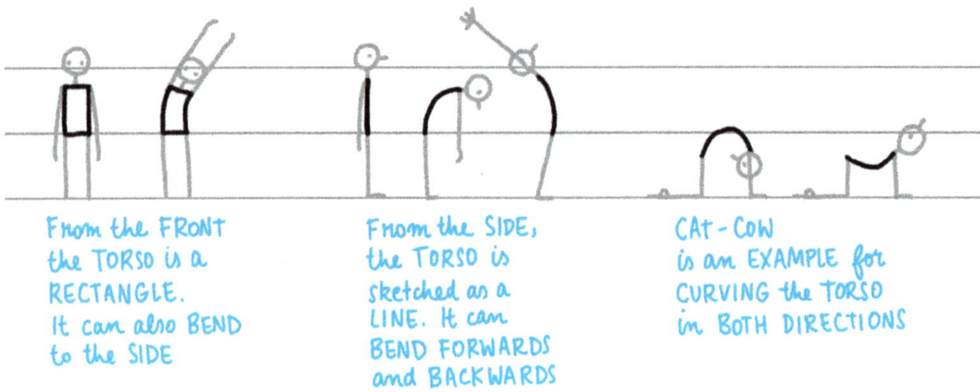

From the FRONT
the TORSO is a
RECTANGLE.
It can also BEND
to the SIDE

From the SIDE,
the TORSO is
sketched as a
LINE. It can
BEND FORWARDS
and BACKWARDS

CAT-COW
is an EXAMPLE for
CURVING the TORSO
in BOTH DIRECTIONS

TWISTING

When the TORSO is TWISTED
from SIDE VIEW (in the LEGS)
to FRONT VIEW (in the CHEST)
we SKETCH it as a TRIANGLE

With this DISTINCTION
we can also SHOW the DIFFERENCE
between EXTENDED & REVOLVED
VERSIONS of the SAME POSE

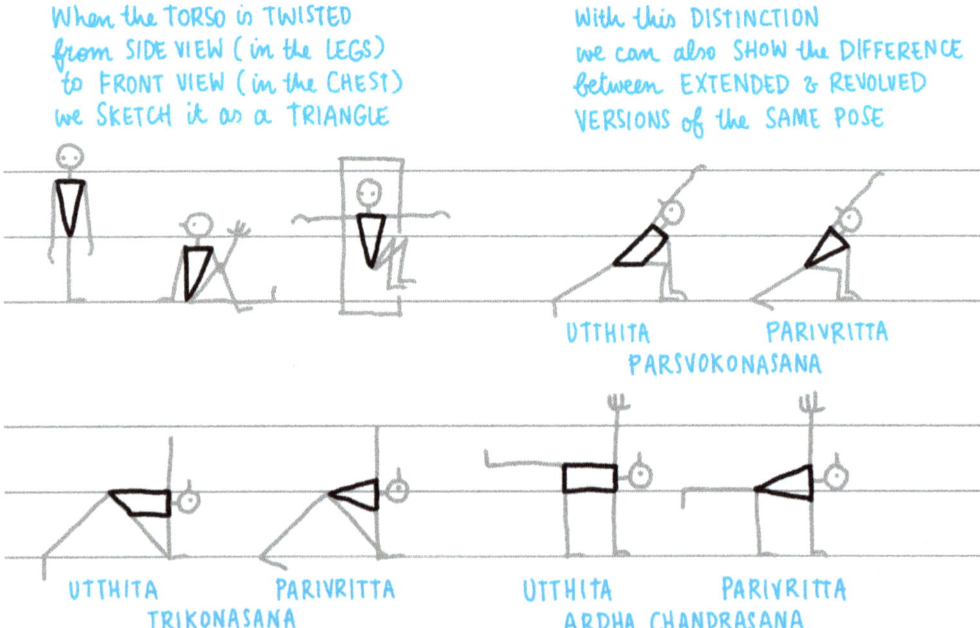

HEAD AND FACE

BASIC HEAD POSITIONS

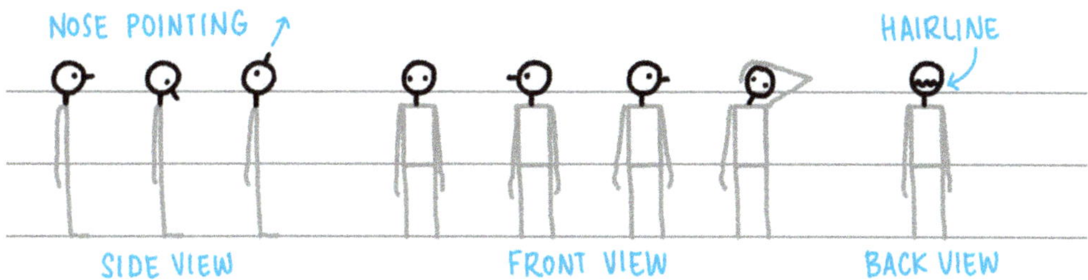

EYE VARIATIONS

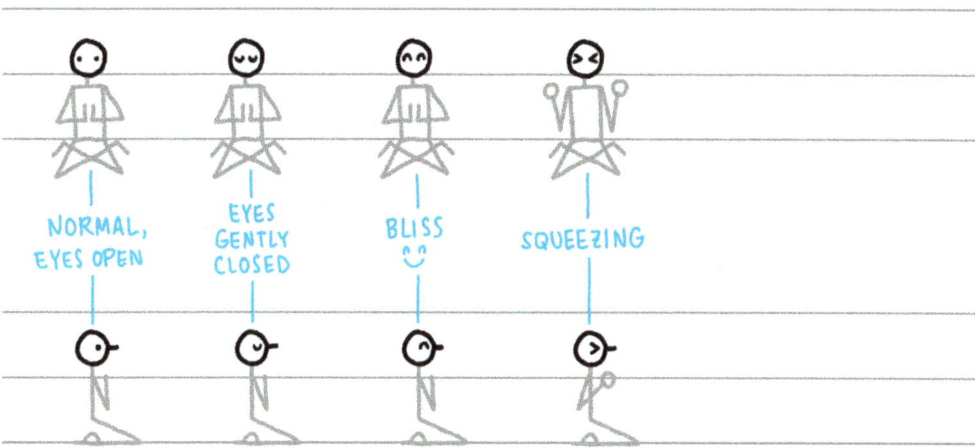

MOVEMENT

There might be occasions when we want to show movement in our sketches: How to enter or exit an asana, moving between two poses (like cat/cow), performing dynamic poses (like leg raises), or flowing through a whole sequence of asanas.

If the movement only involves one part of the body while the rest stays relatively static, we can sketch the changed position of the moving part on top of the basic pose and indicate the movement between the two states with an arrow.

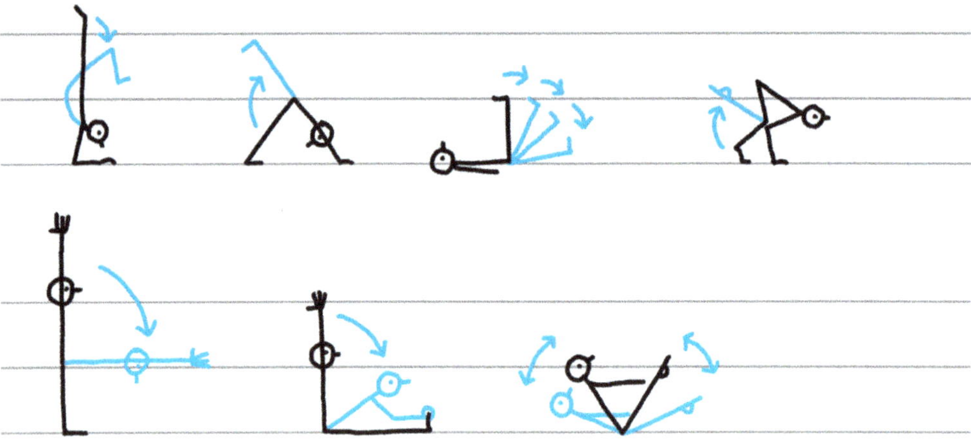

If the movement involves changing most of the body position, it is better to sketch the start and end position as separate sketches and to connect the two sketches with arrows. We can also add notes on the number of repetitions.

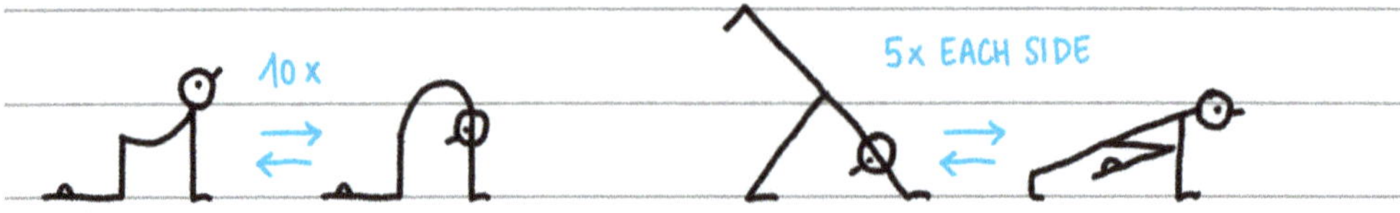

To show a sequence of movements in detail, we can break down
the movement into different steps and describe the movement for
each step by using arrows and short descriptions.

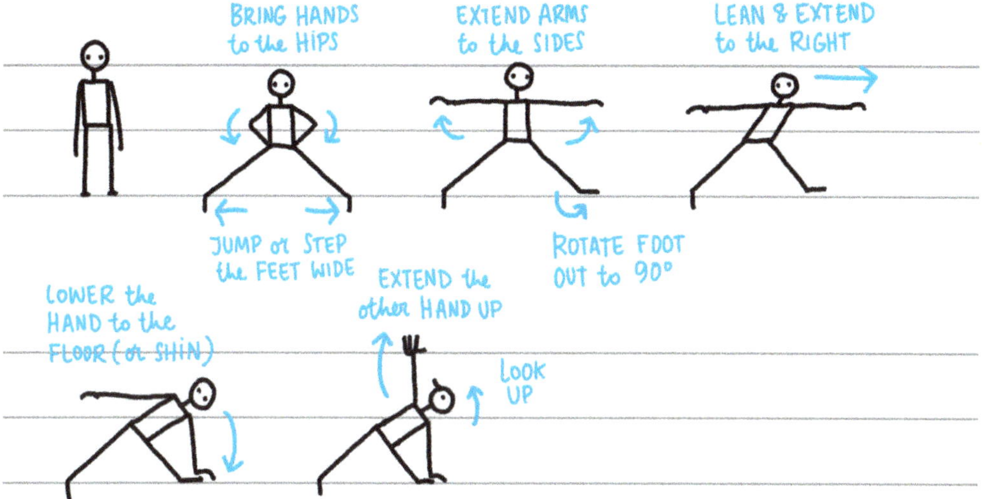

The best way to keep clarity while adding movement is to use a
second colour. Thanks to our visual perception, we naturally see
different colours as separate layers of information.

If you don't have a second colour handy, you can use dotted lines
instead. It is less clear than a second colour, but still provides
enough visual distinction.

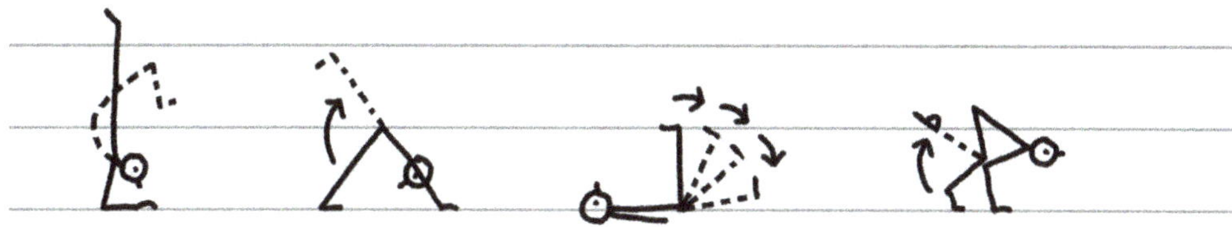

PROPS

Using props like blocks, bolsters and straps is a great way to modify postures for beginners, when we are stiff or are recovering from an injury.

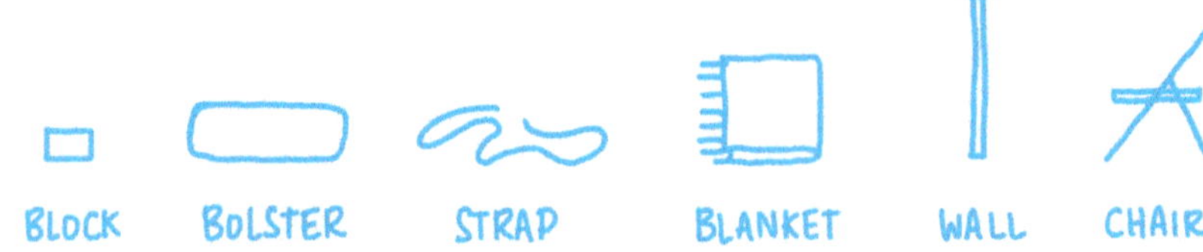

I like to sketch props in a different colour, so they look clearly different from the figure and it's easy to see where they are placed.

BLOCKS

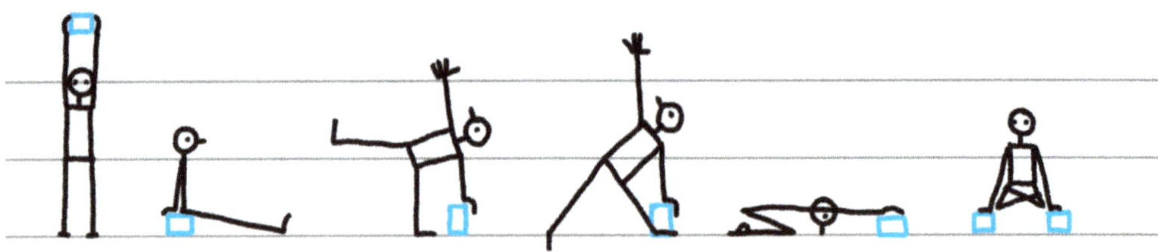

STRAPS

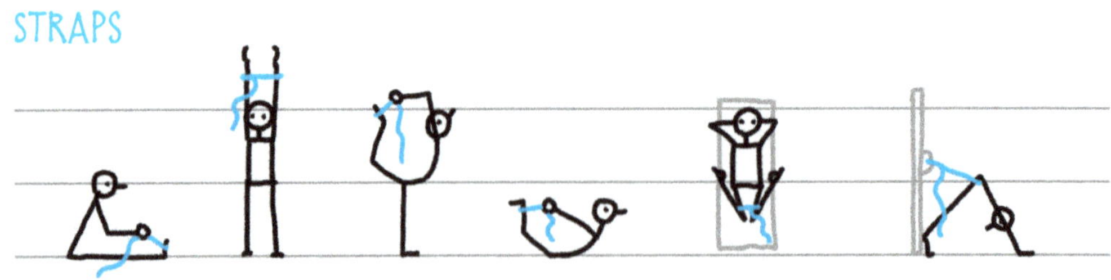

BOLSTERS

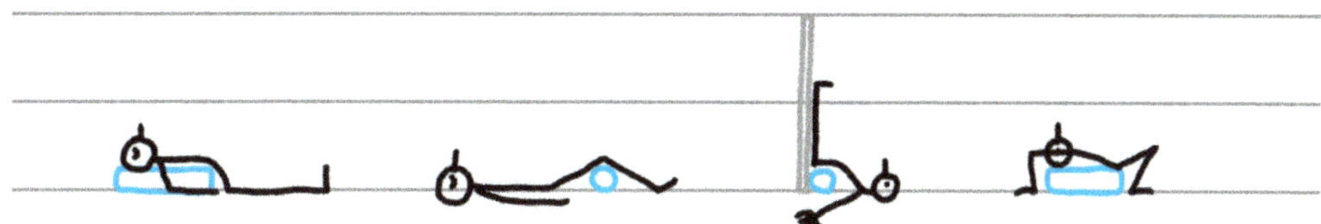

BLANKETS

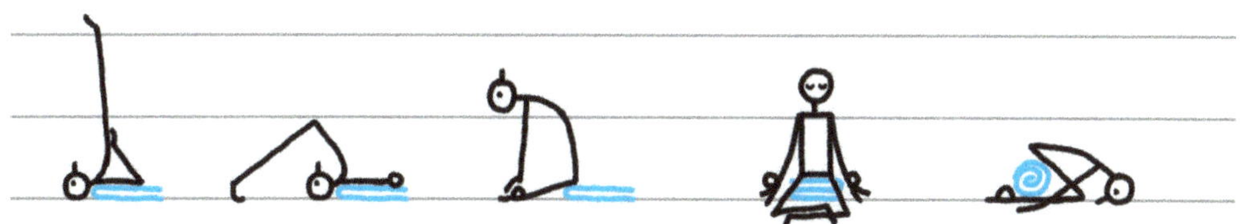

WALL

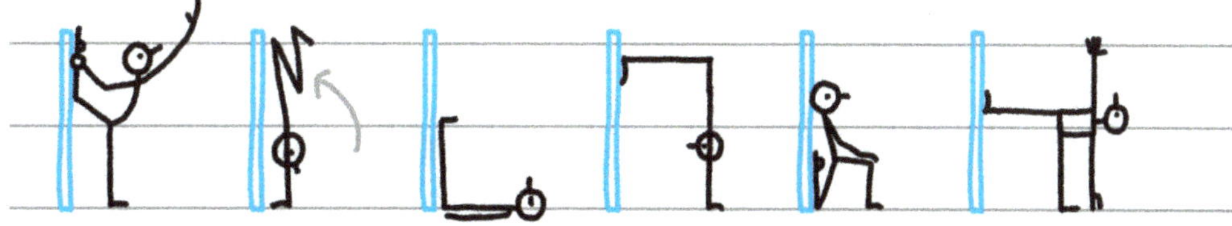

CHAIR

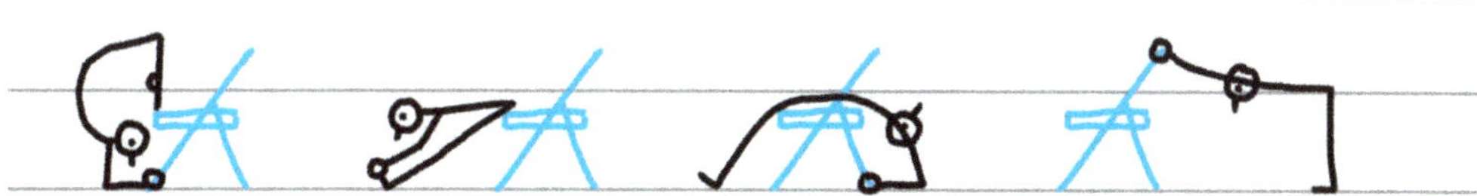

ANNOTATIONS

So far we have been focussing on how to create the visual
part of our sketches. But there is an equally important part that
complements the drawings: language. Words and visuals are
perfect partners for conveying information.

We can use words to describe the more subtle aspects of the
asana that can't necessarily be seen, like muscle tension, rotation,
or focus.

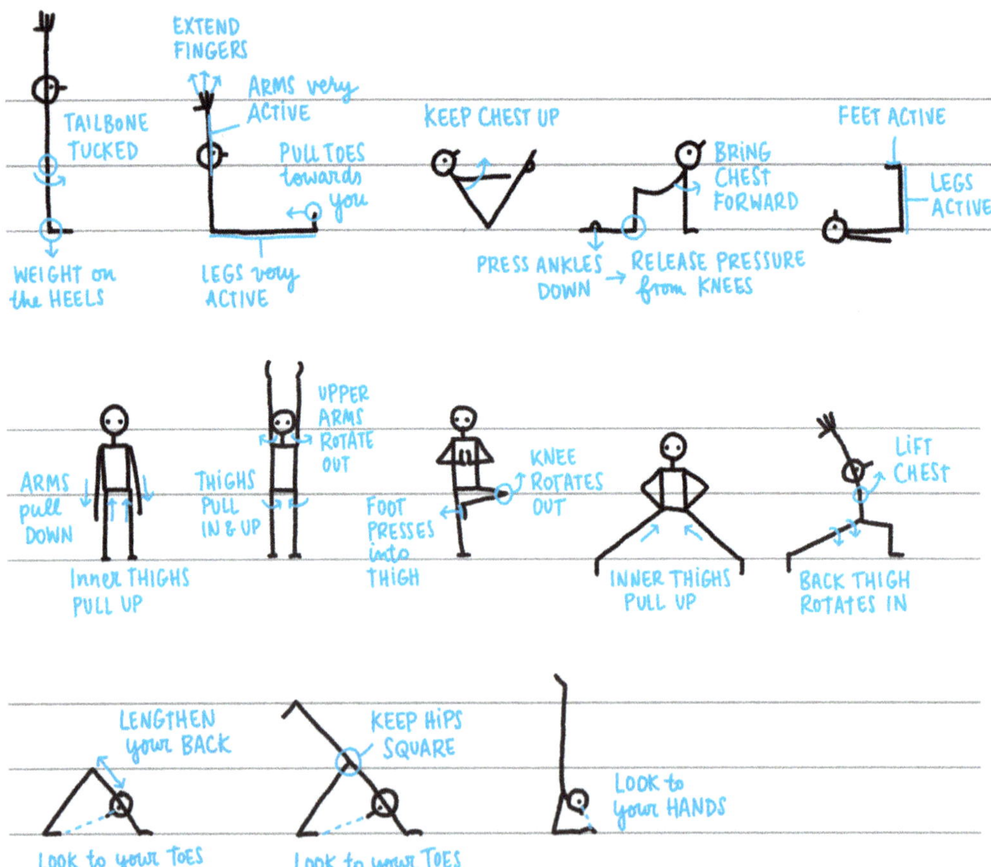

We can add notes on breath, how long to hold a posture, or write
down the cues we want to give in class.

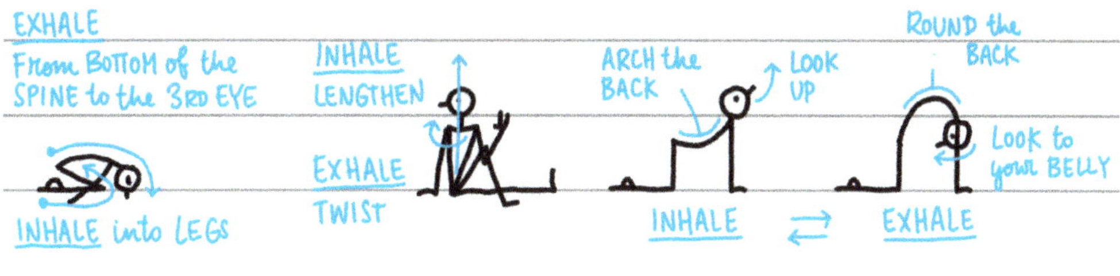

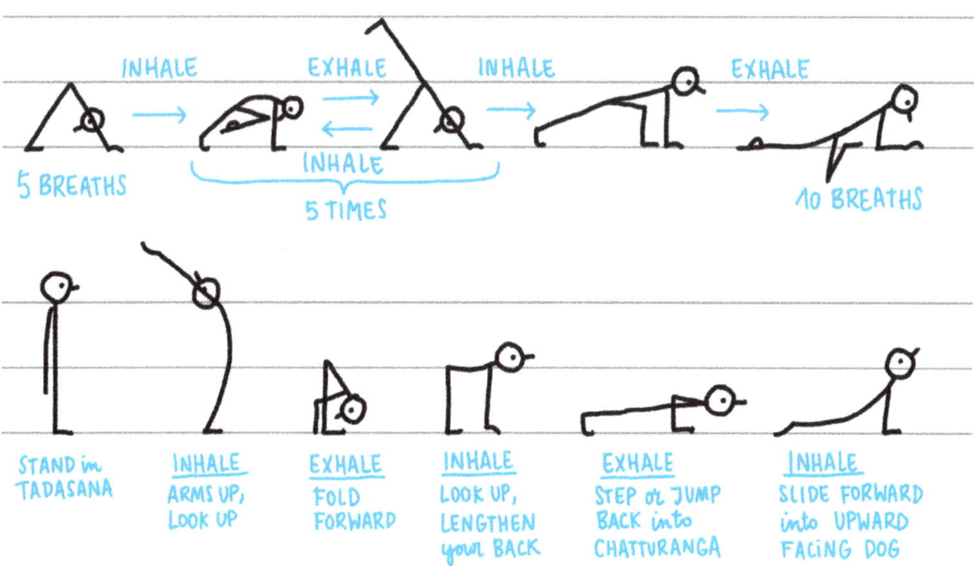

I always use a different colour for my annotations. This allows
me to circle or mark any part of the figure without reducing the
readability of the sketch. Our eyes naturally perceive different
colours as different layers of information. Even when we add a lot
of text, the sketches underneath are still clearly visible and easy to
follow at a glance.

PUTTING TOGETHER SEQUENCES

After learning the basics and a bit of practice sketching individual asanas, you can start putting together whole sequences.

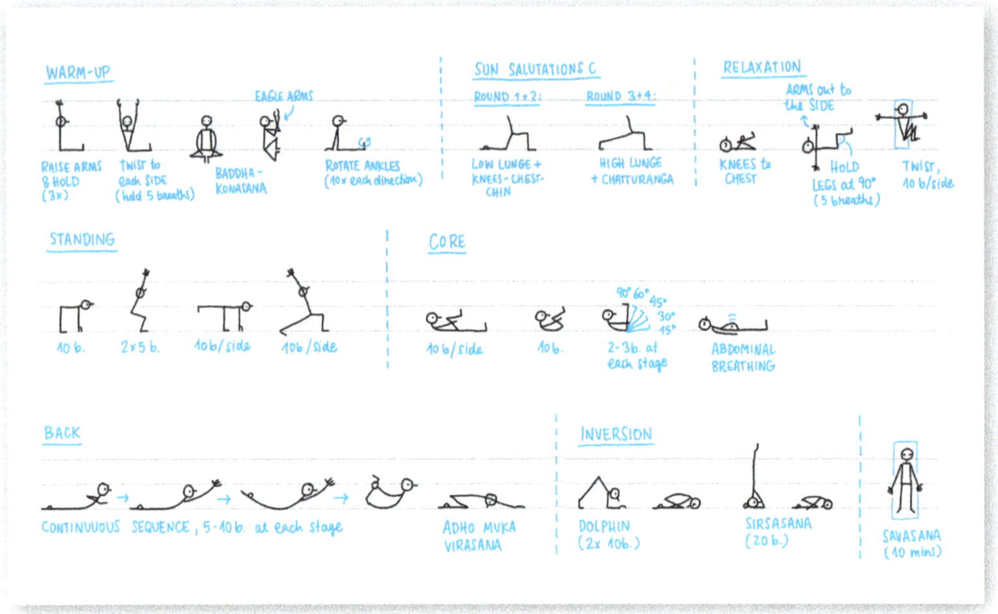

I like creating visual overviews of my favourite sequences so I can go through them before I practice or look at the sheet from my mat during practice when I get a bit lost. These sheets are perfect to use for self-practice when you travel, can't attend class or have no internet connection to stream a class online.

Sketching out sequences is also a great way for teachers to plan a class. Instead of just writing down a list of posture names, you can visualise the flow of the class while you plan it – making it easy to bring the right types of asanas together and to create a balanced sequence.

You can also make copies of your sketched sequence as hand-outs or home-practice guides for your students.

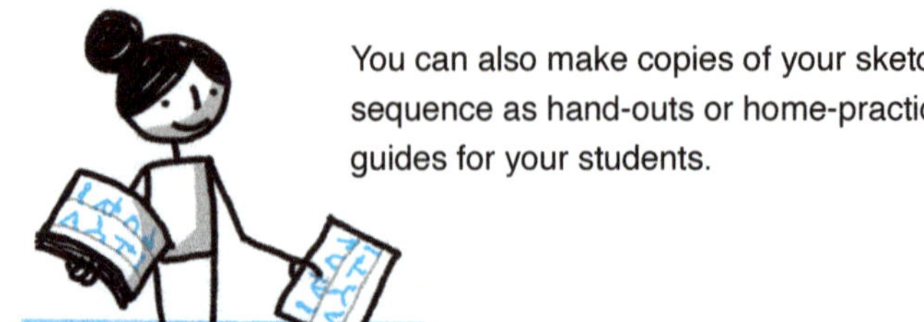

Sketching a sequence is pretty straight forward. We just sketch one posture after the other, leaving enough space inbetween to add our annotations on movement, alignment, breathing or timing later.

We can also sketch an asana, add the annotations straight away and then move on to sketch the next posture. Like that we don't run out of space when we write our notes for each posture.

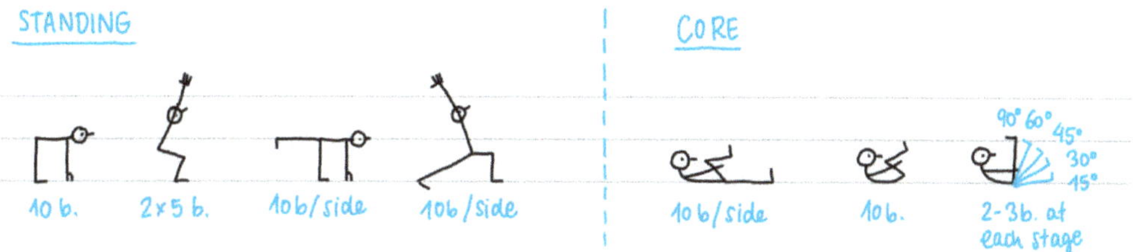

For postures or whole sequences that are performed on both sides (like Trikonasana, or Surya Namaskar B), I only sketch them once, noting which side to start with (we start with the right side in most postures) and marking which part of the sequence needs to be repeated on the other side.

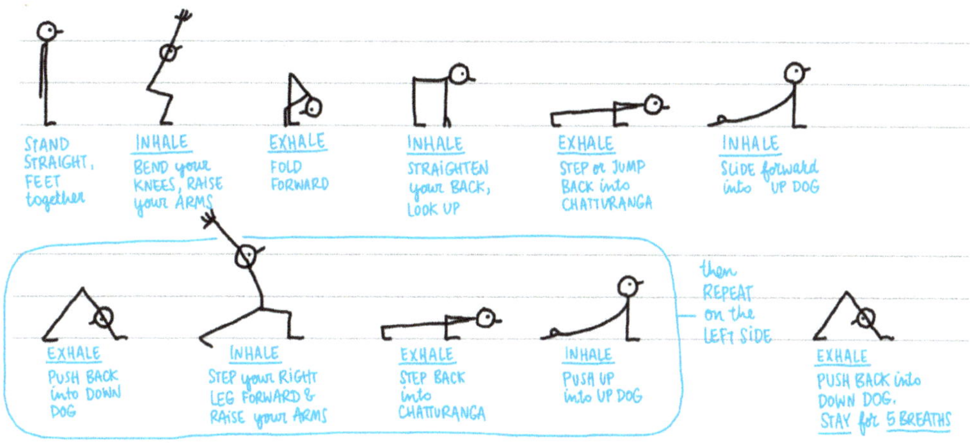

When planning a new sequence, the
process can be a bit messy at first: sketching
some postures, crossing them out again,
adding in postures, or rearranging whole
parts with arrows as the sequence takes
shape. That's totally fine and a great working
process.

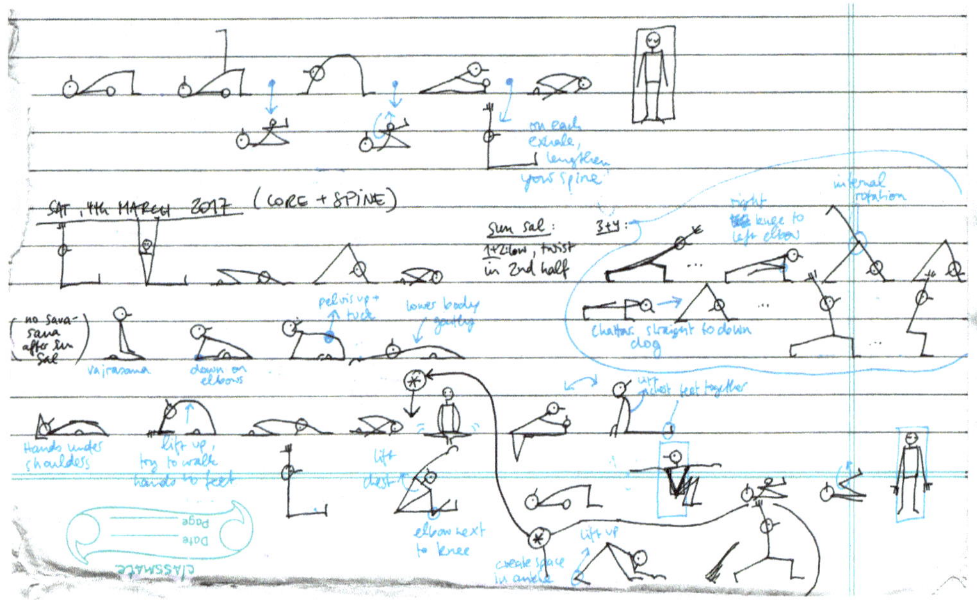

Once we have finished planning and
we're happy with the flow, we just take a
fresh sheet of paper and draw the whole
sequence again.

In part 3, you will find sketched sample
sequences (3 Sun Salutations and a
complete Hatha class).

PENS AND PAPER

You don't need any special pens or paper to
start sketching. My motto is:
"Any pen is better than no pen."

Try out different pens, and over time you will
find your favourites. Here are a few thoughts
on how I pick my pens.

NO ERASERS

I like to use pens that can't be erased.
Sketching is about making marks, not about
taking them away. If I make a wrong line, I
just put the correct line right on top. If there
are too many wrong lines, I cross out the
sketch and make a new one.

When I have the option to erase, I often get
hung up in my quest for perfection, erasing
and re-erasing a single line over and over.
Not giving myselves the option to erase,
helps me to not fall into this trap.

It might feel uncomfortable at first, but over
time, we build more confidence in our work if
we commit to our lines, even if they are not
perfect.

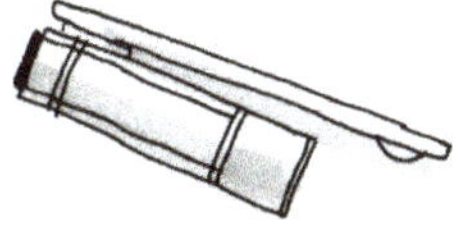

THE RIGHT THICKNESS

I usually use a regular black fineliner or gel
pen to sketch my asanas. As I sketch rather
small, I like thinner pens, so I still have
enough clarity even in a small space.
Try out a few pens of different thicknesses to
find the one that is right for you. In general,
a bit thinner is better than too thick.

COLOURS

As I explained in the previous chapters,
having one or two extra colours is great to
add movement, props or annotations.
I use coloured fineliners similar to my main
black pen. The colours I choose are bright
and vivid, so they contrast nicely with the
black, but also dark enough to be readable.
I usually go for orange, a nice cyan blue or
apple green.

PAPER

In terms of paper, I am not particularly picky.
Just simple A4 or Letter sized printer paper
is fine. I like to print out my own guidelines
as they help me to sketch the asanas in
proportion and to keep them nicely lined up.

You can download my printable templates
on my website: **www.yoganotes.net**

You can also use any lined paper or
notebook. Mark every 6th line as a baseline
and you'll have enough space between the
lines to fit the postures and your notes.

And with a little bit of practice you can even
sketch without any guidelines at all.

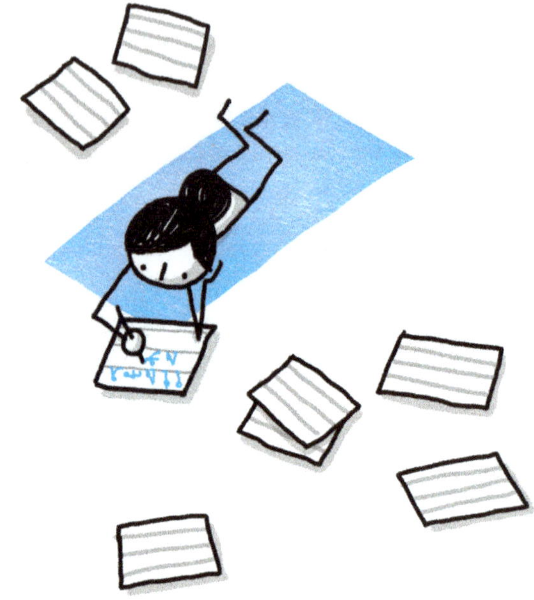

ONE LAST TIP

Whatever material you use and prefer,
make sure that you don't get depended
on it. Not having your favourite pens and
notebook with you should never be a
reason not to sketch.

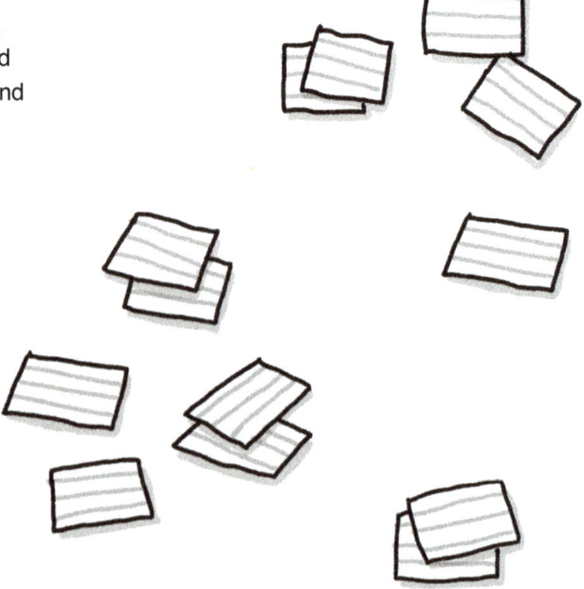

MAKE YOUR OWN YOGA AVATAR

After all the hard work we've been doing so far, it is time to have a little fun. We can use everything we learnt so far to create our own little yoga avatars (and maybe some for our friends, too!). Choose your favourite yoga pose and sketch it. But instead of sketching the head at the normal size, make it much bigger. Then personalise it with your own features: Hairstyle, facial expressions, glasses or even a beard.

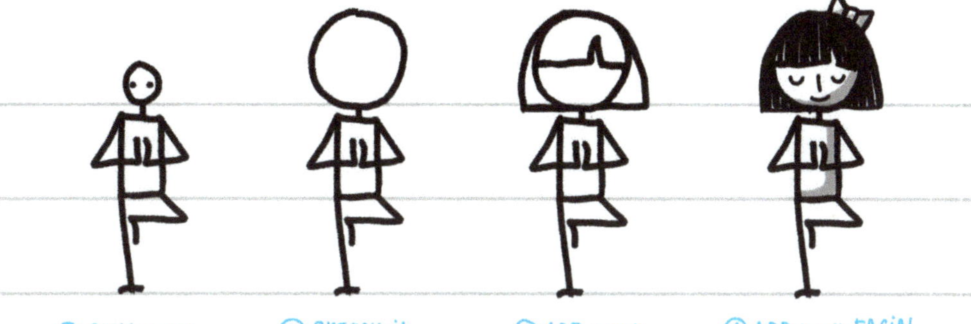

① PICK your FAVOURITE YOGA POSE

② SKETCH it with a very BIG HEAD

③ ADD your HAIR STYLE

④ ADD your FACIAL FEATURES and any ACCESSORIES.

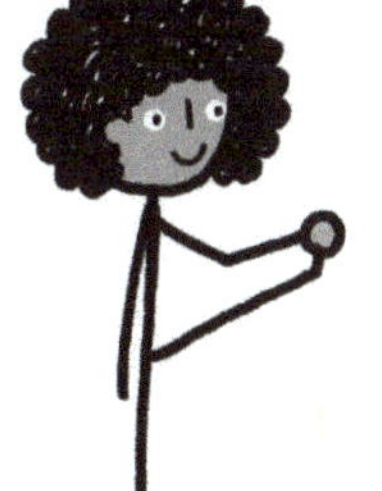

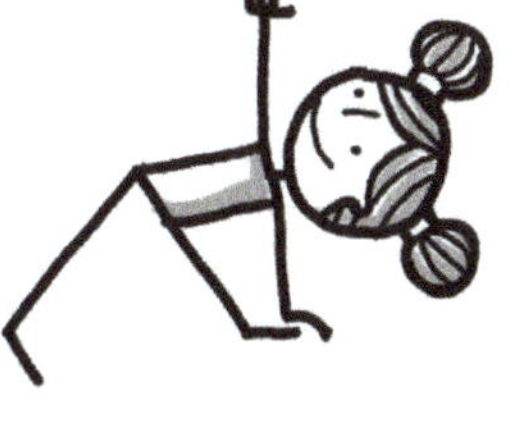

If you would like to learn all about creating your own Yoga-Avatar and get lots of inspiration for how to draw hairstyles, clothes and accessories, check out my e-book 'Draw your Yoga-Avatar':

WWW. EVALOTTA.SHOP/ YOGAAVATAR

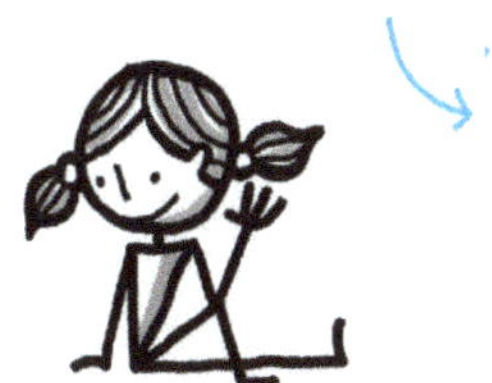

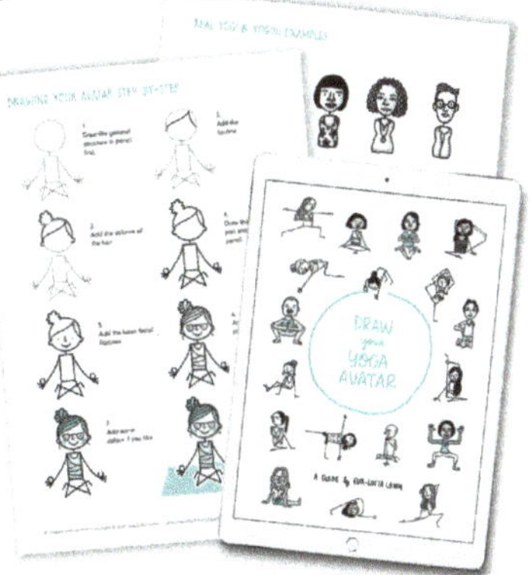

SHARE YOUR WORK

Before we close this chapter and move on to the step-by-step asana instructions, I want to encourage you to share your work. We grow by sharing what we know and by being inspired by what others share with us.

In a community, everybody is a valued contributor and by opening up and sharing our thoughts, ideas and our work, we can connect with others, build relationships and support each other.

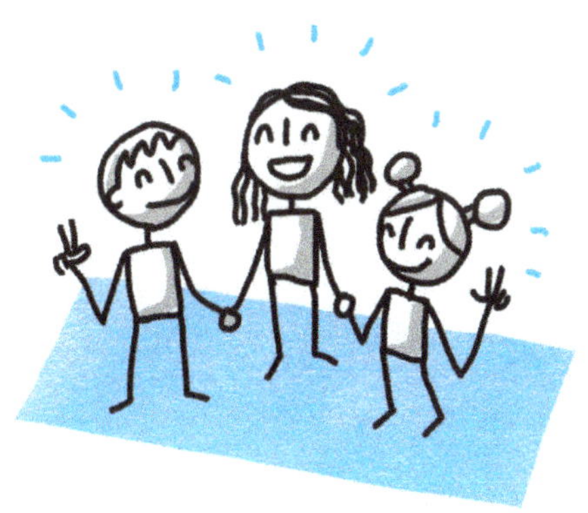

Your sketches don't have to be perfect. They are great as they are. We all start somewhere and it is beautiful and inspiring to see somebody's journey from the very beginning. So please, do share your sketches with the world and let's all learn and grow together.

If you post your sketches on Instagram, use the hashtag #yoganotes to add them to the community. You can also tag me as @yoga. notes so I can find your work. I can't wait to see what you will create.

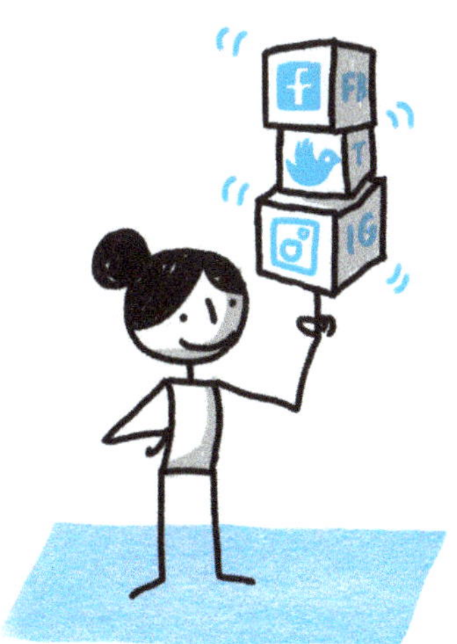

CONNECT WITH THE YOGANOTES COMMUNITY

Hashtag: #yoganotes
Instagram: @yoga.notes
Facebook: sketchyoganotes
Web: www.yoganotes.net

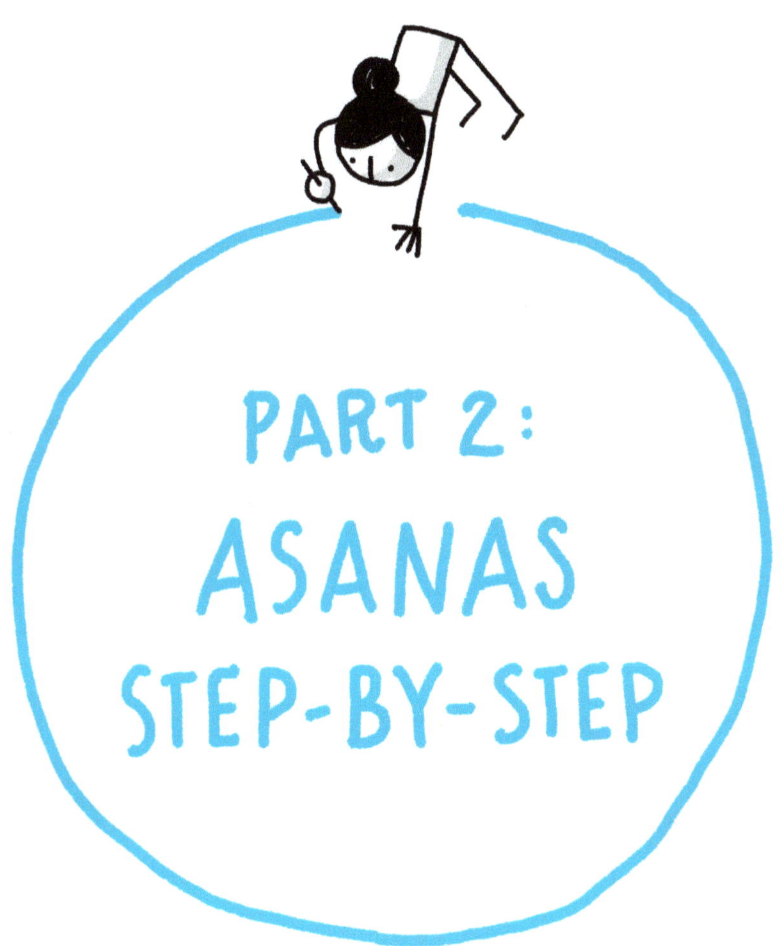

PART 2:
ASANAS
STEP-BY-STEP

ASANAS - STEP BY STEP

In this part of the book you will find step-by-step instructions for over 80 asanas, including variations, modifications and preparatory steps to enter a pose.

Each sheet lists the Sanskrit and the English name. On the right, you find the keywords for categorising the pose in several ways (standing, sitting, forward bend, restorative, etc.).

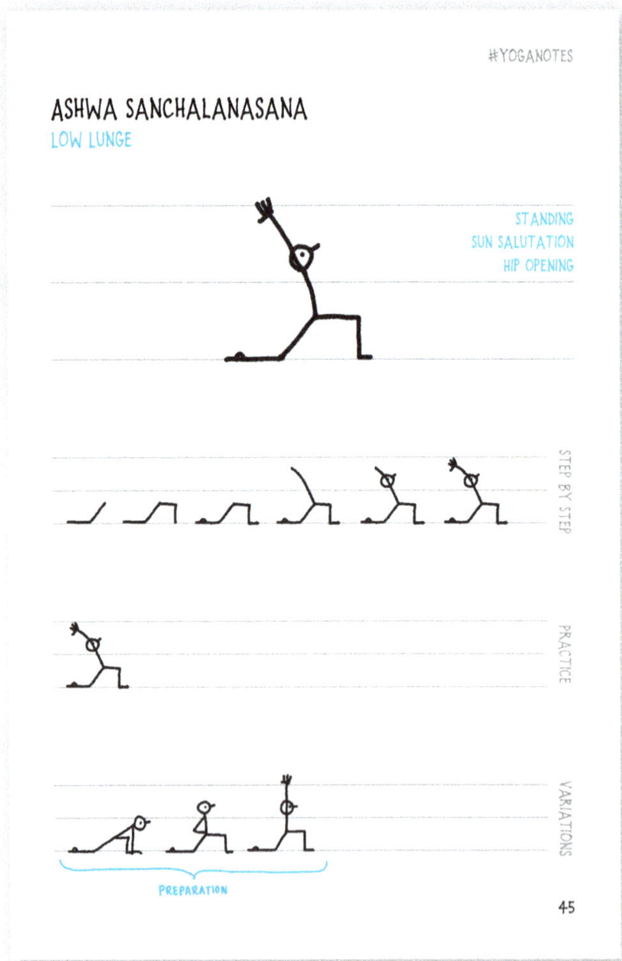

For each asana there is one big sketch, so you can see every detail nicely and clearly.

Next, there are step-by-step instructions. You can follow along sketching each stroke in the right order.

Below is your practice area, where you sketch the pose yourself. Once you filled the practice area you can print out more blank lined templates (see page 34 for the link) to repeat each pose until you master it.

The last section contains variations and modifications of the pose. For some poses the preparatory steps to get into the pose are shown.

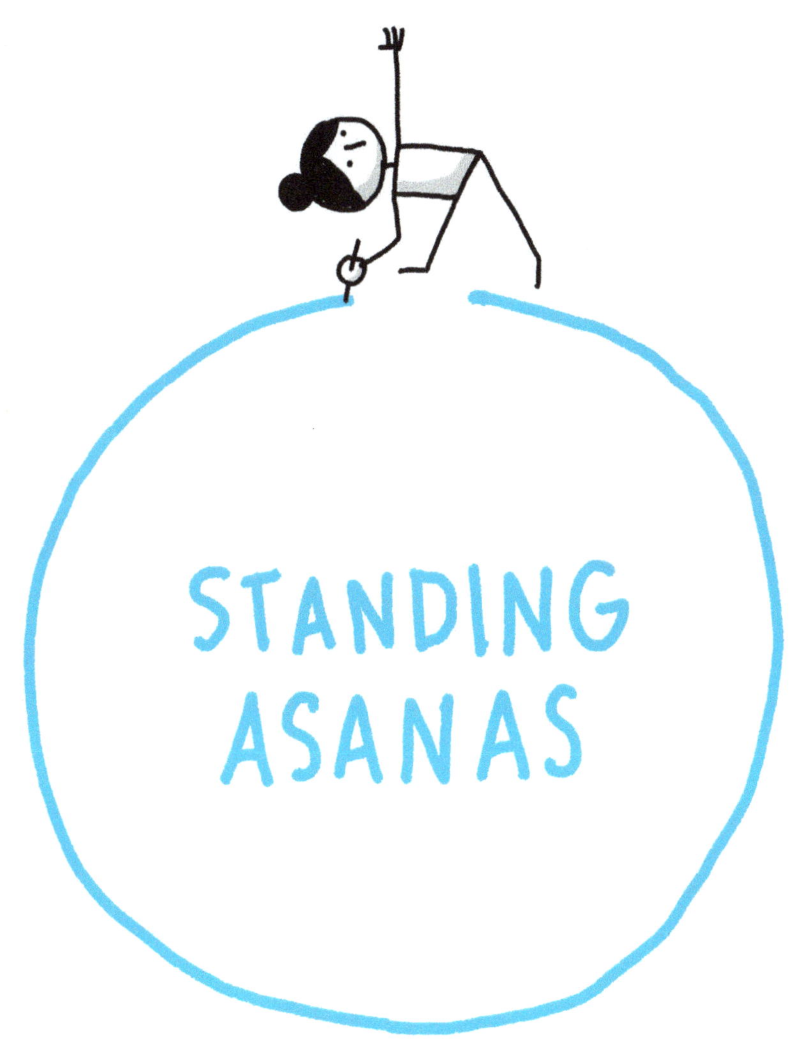

STANDING
ASANAS

TADASANA
MOUNTAIN POSE

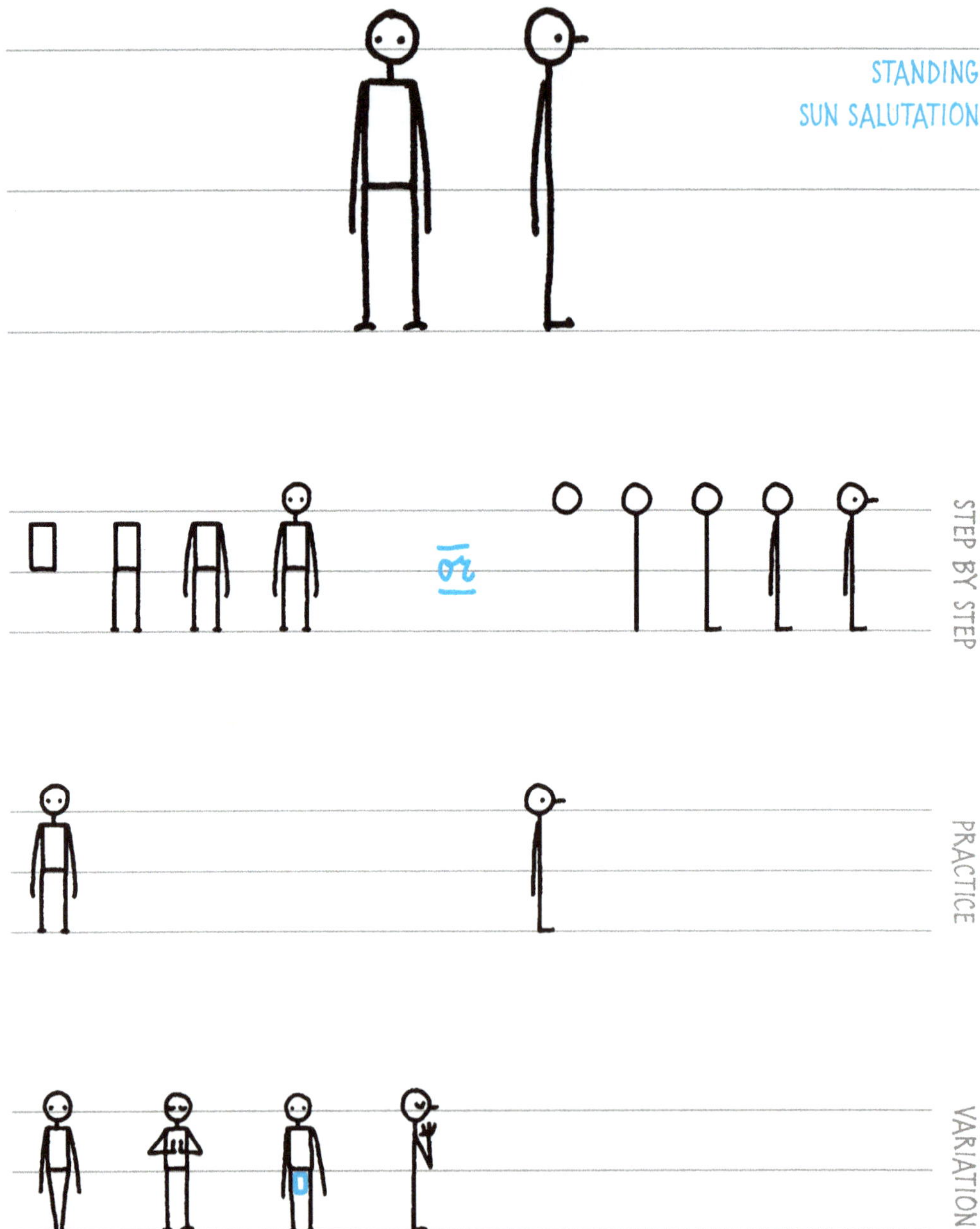

URDHVA HASTASANA

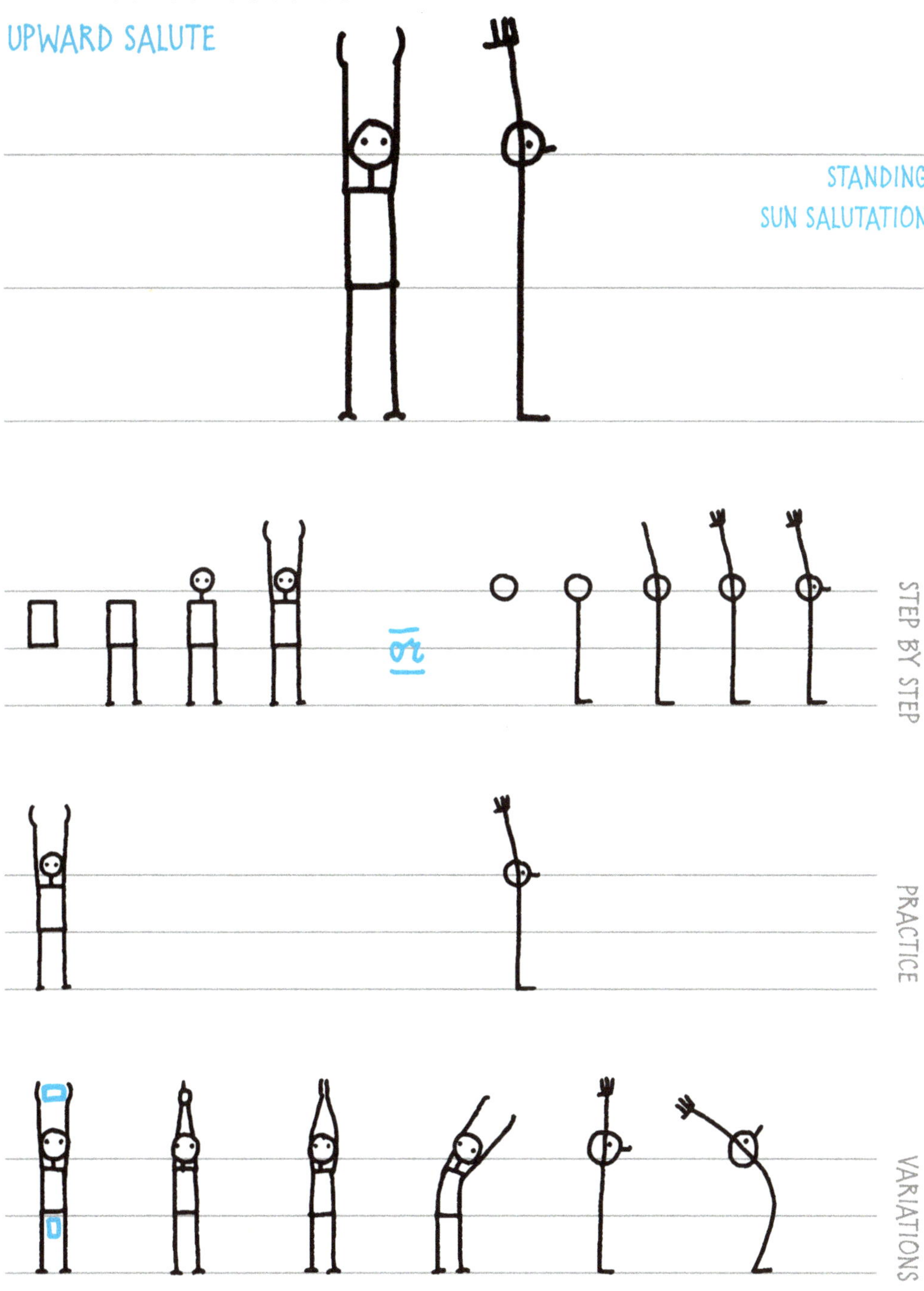

UTTANASANA
STANDING FORWARD FOLD

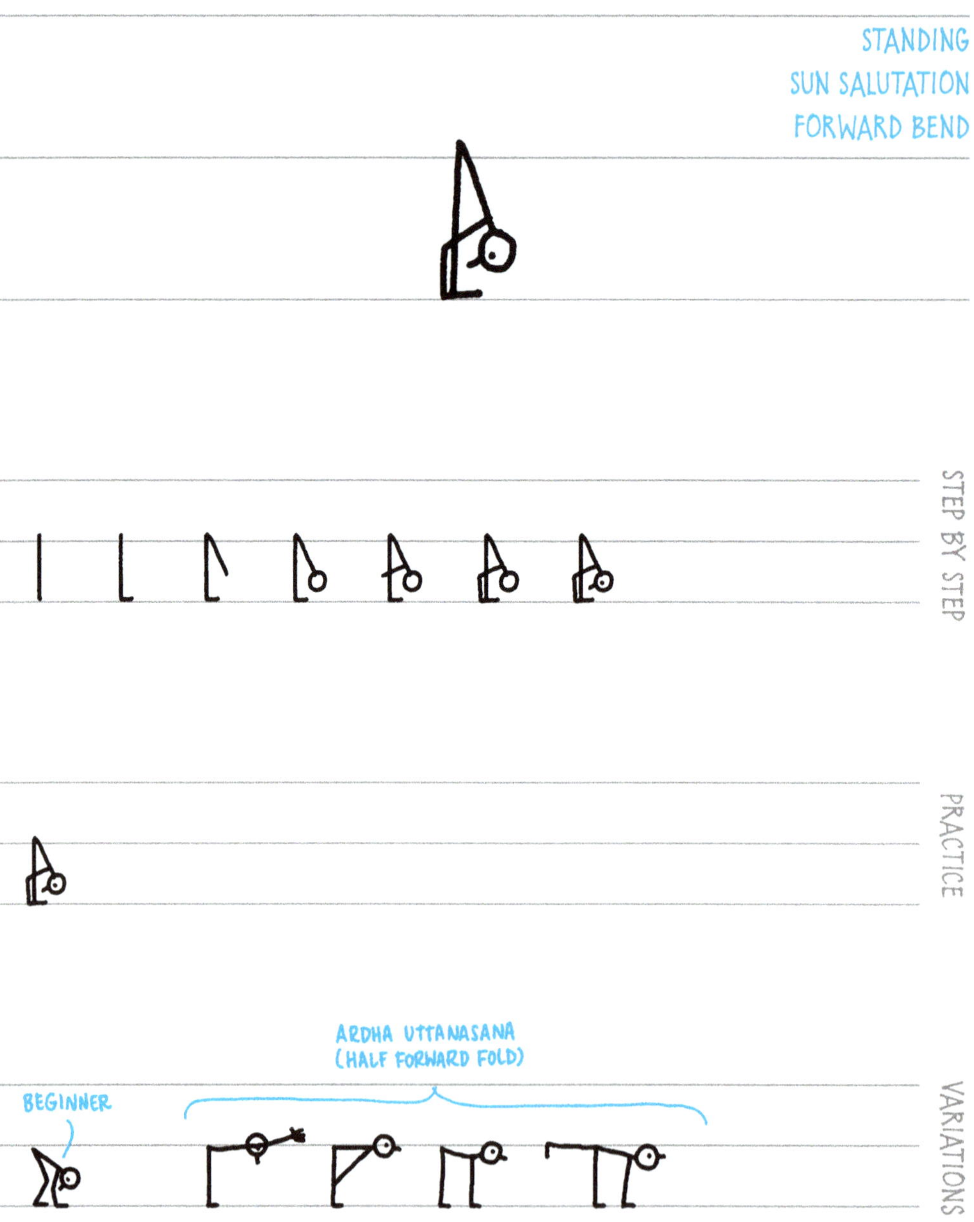

ASHWA SANCHALANASANA

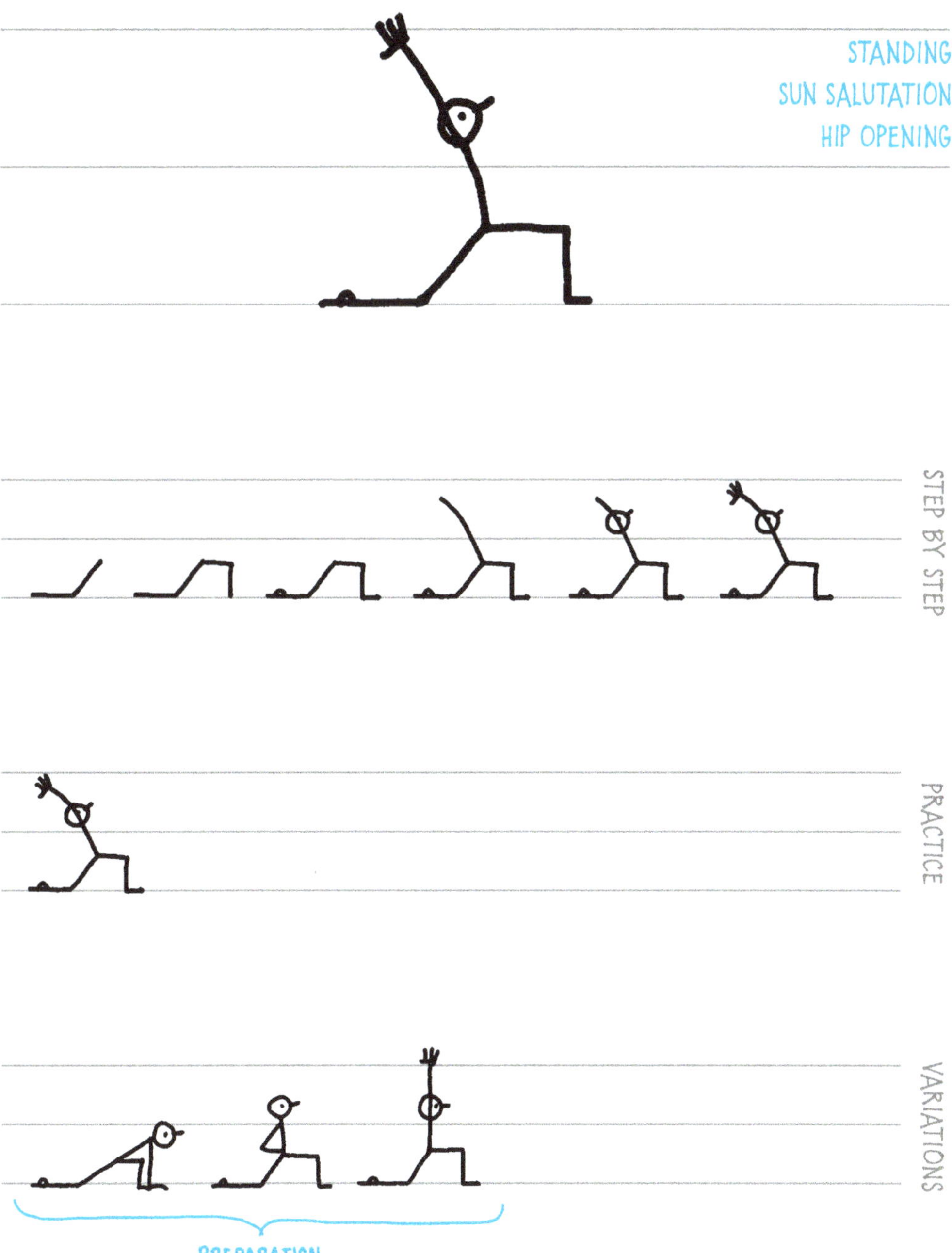

UTTHITA ASHWA SANCHALANASANA
HIGH LUNGE

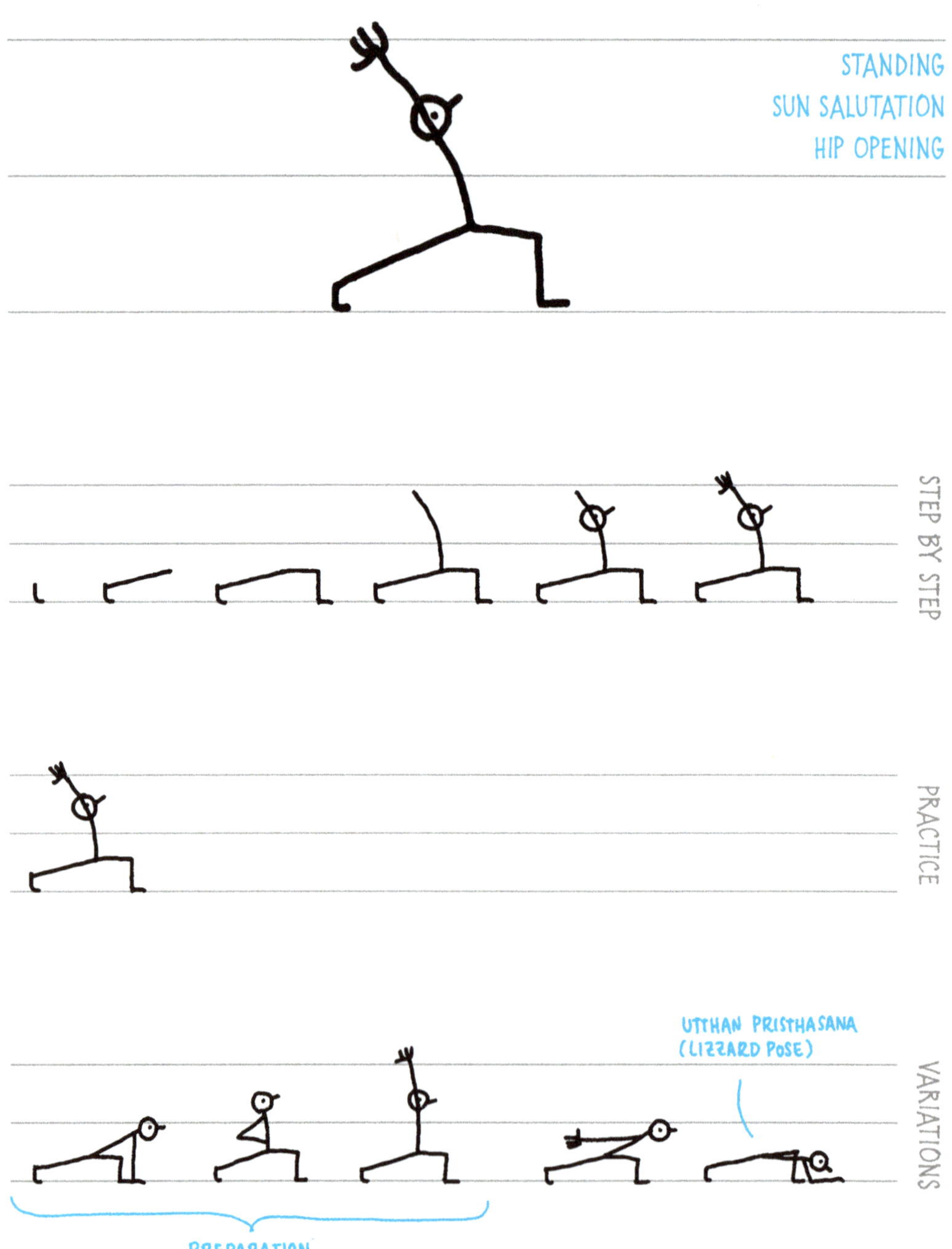

ADHO MUKHA SVANASANA

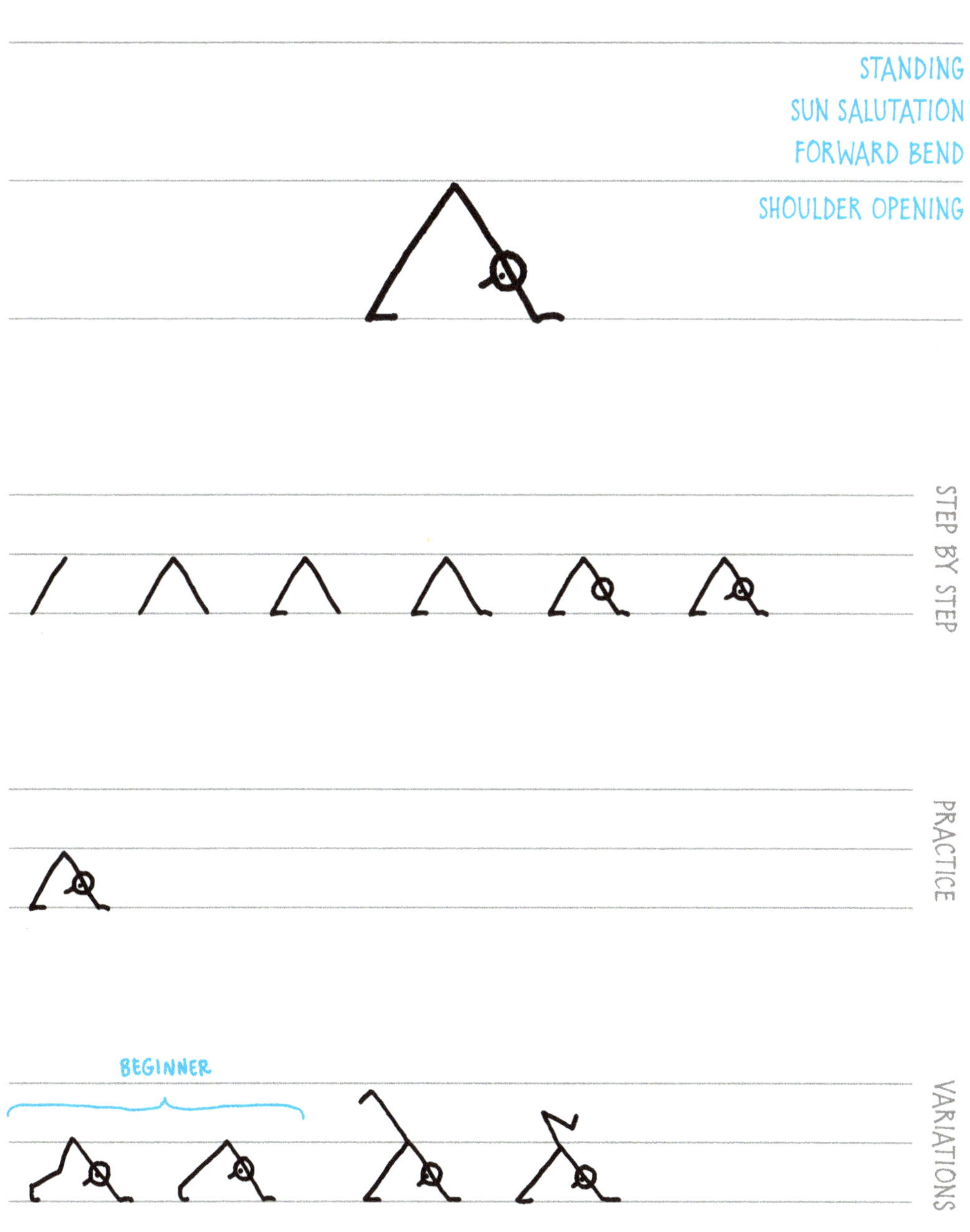

VIRABHADRASANA I

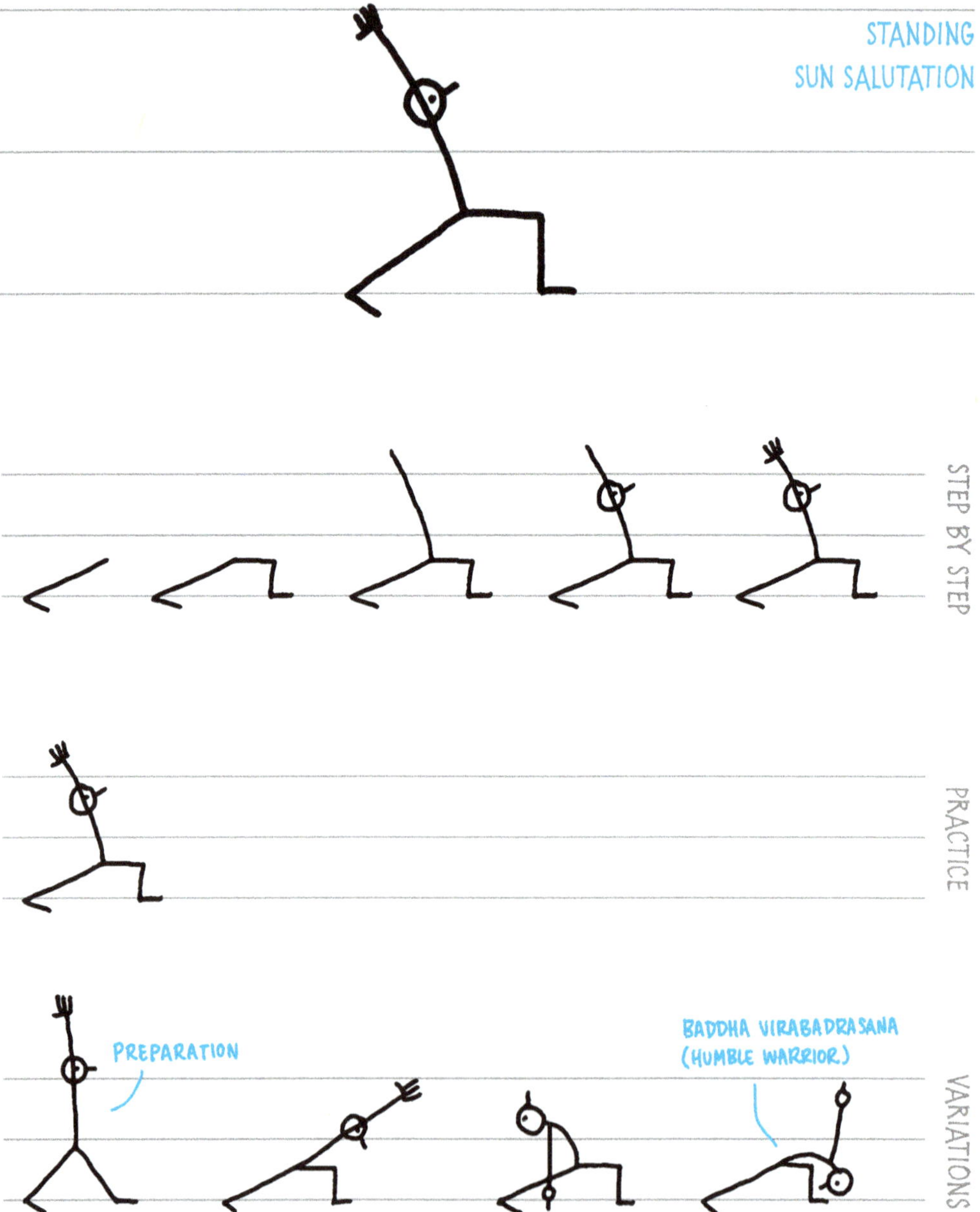

VIRABHADRASANA II

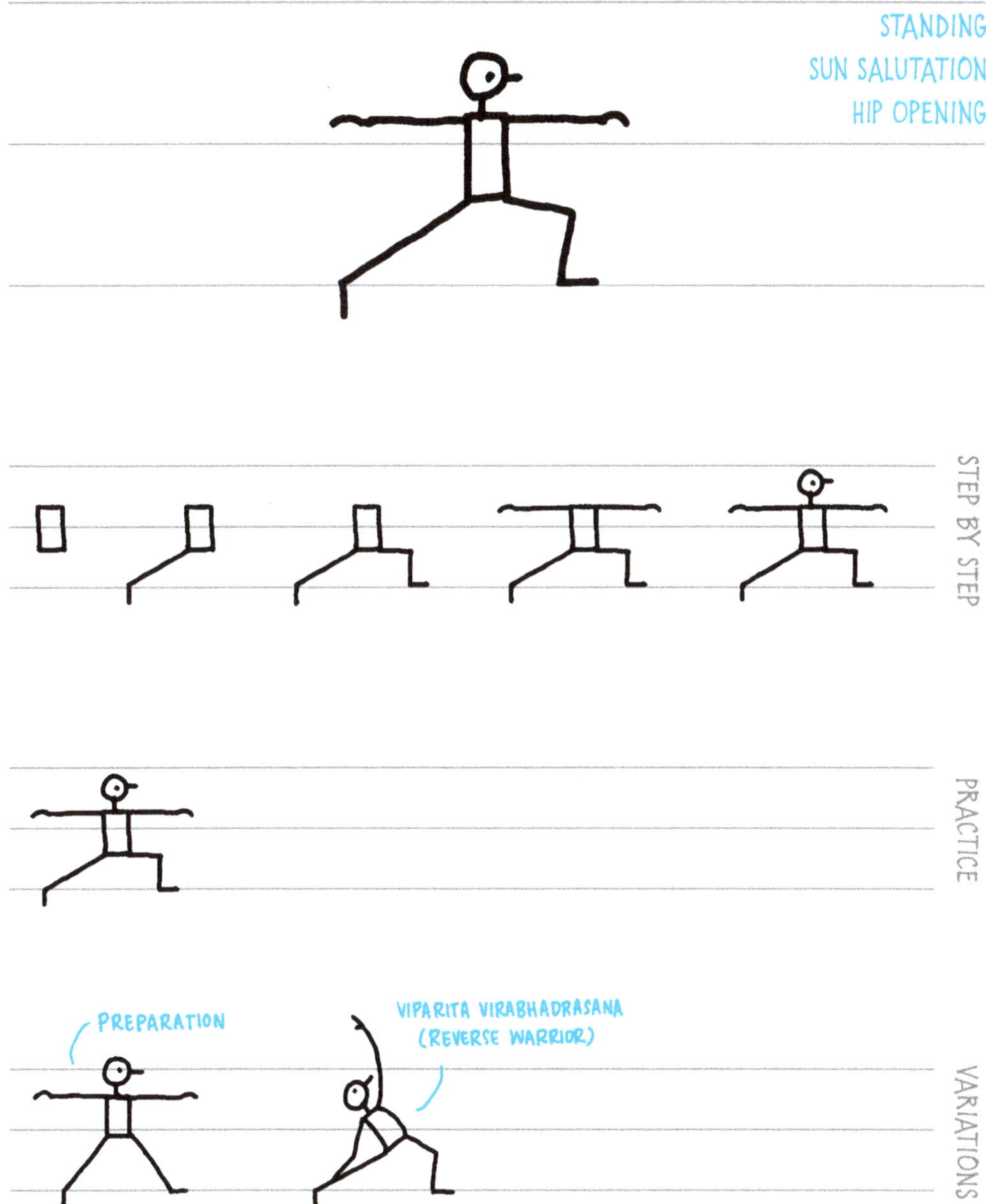

VIRABHADRASANA III

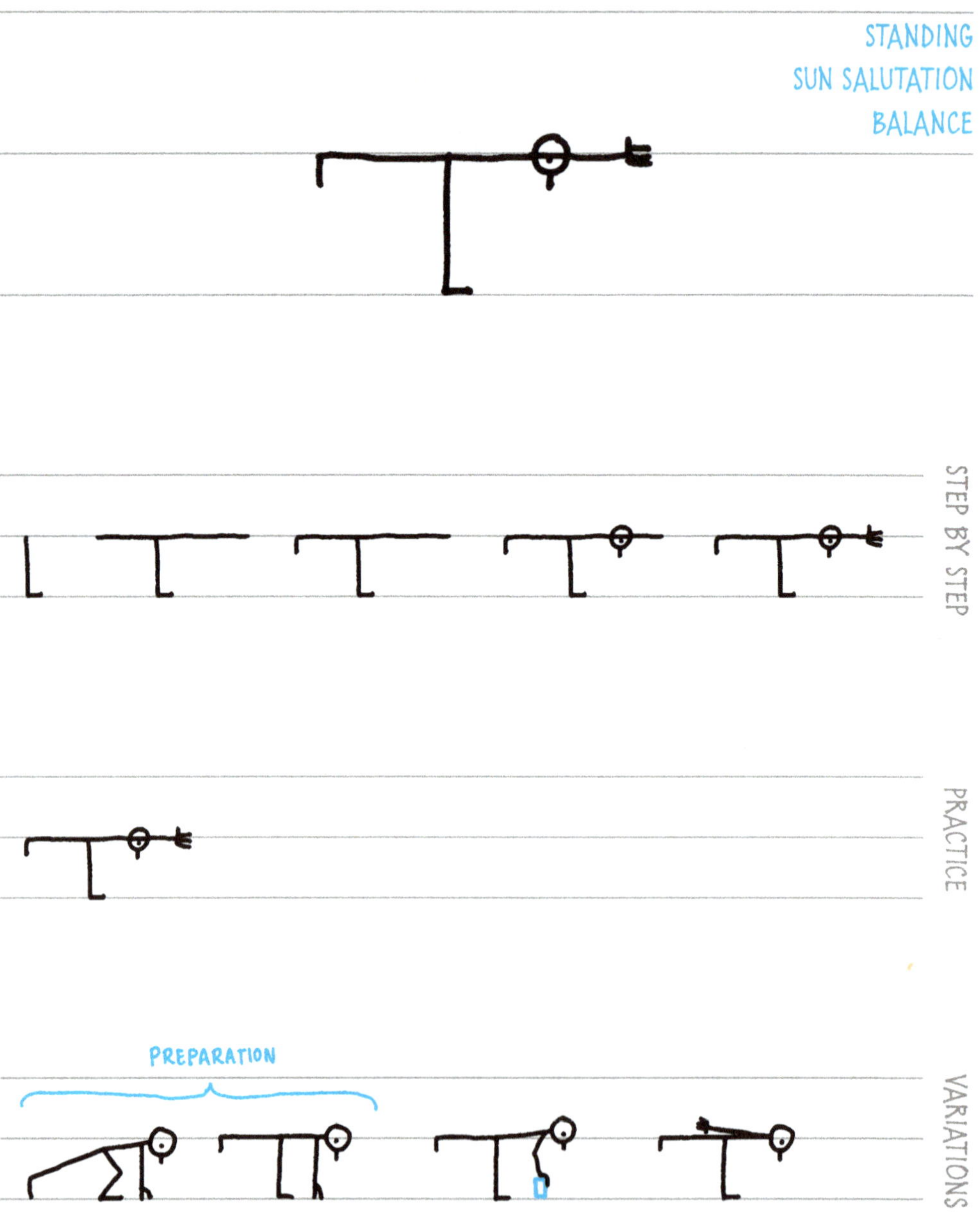

UTTHITA PARSVAKONASANA I
EXTENDED SIDE ANGLE POSE

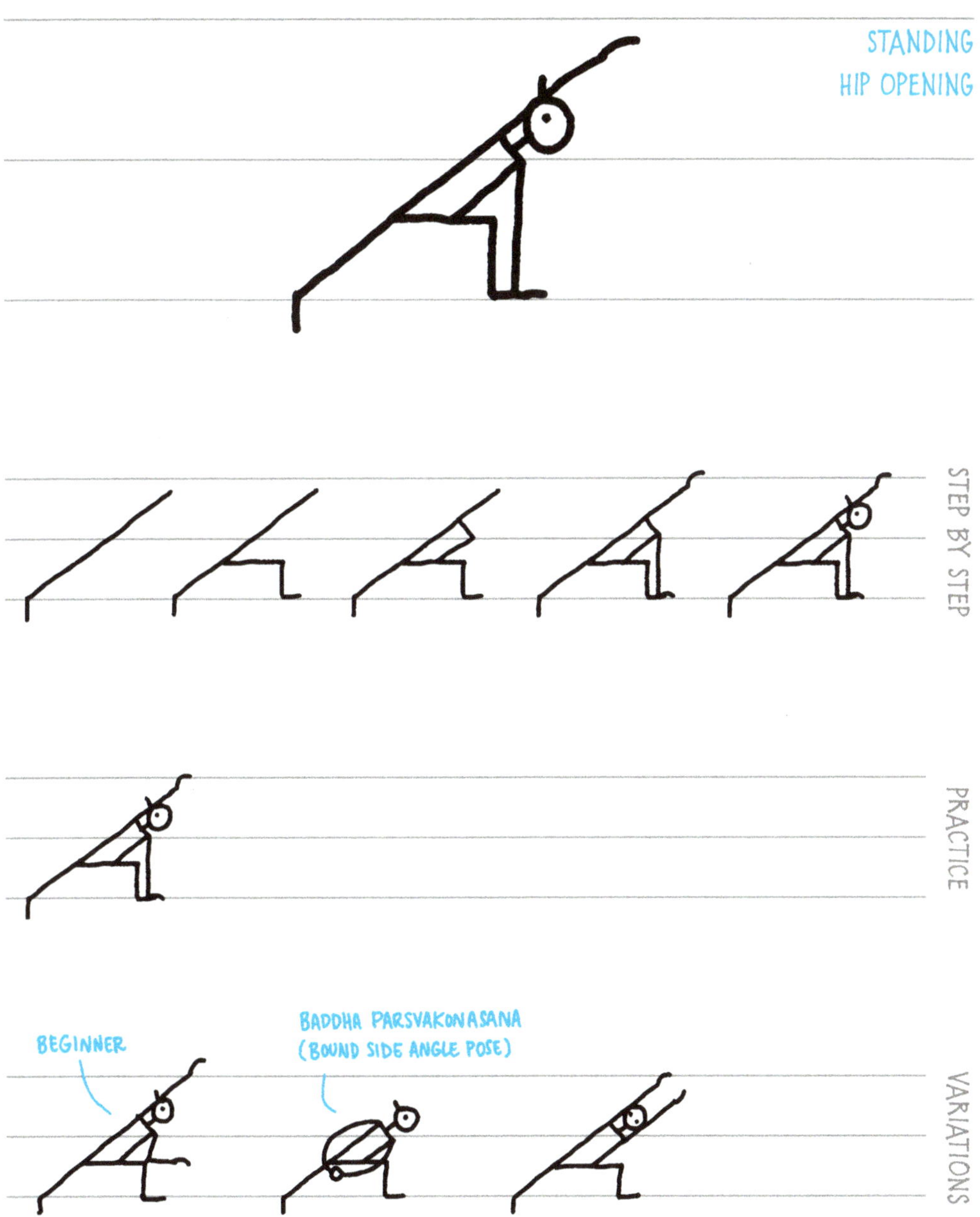

PARIVRTTA PARSVAKONASANA
REVOLVED SIDE ANGLE POSE

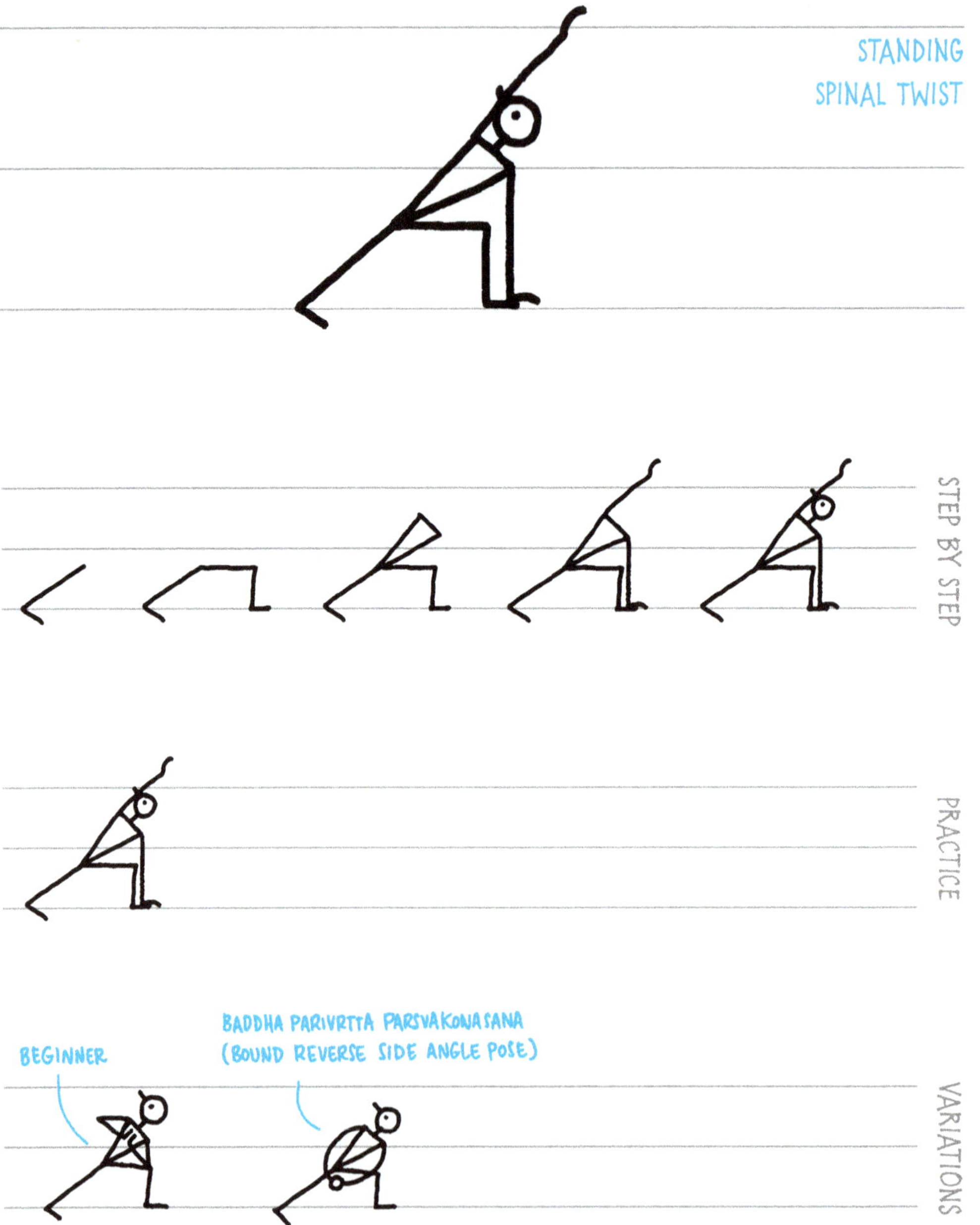

SVARGA DVIJASANA

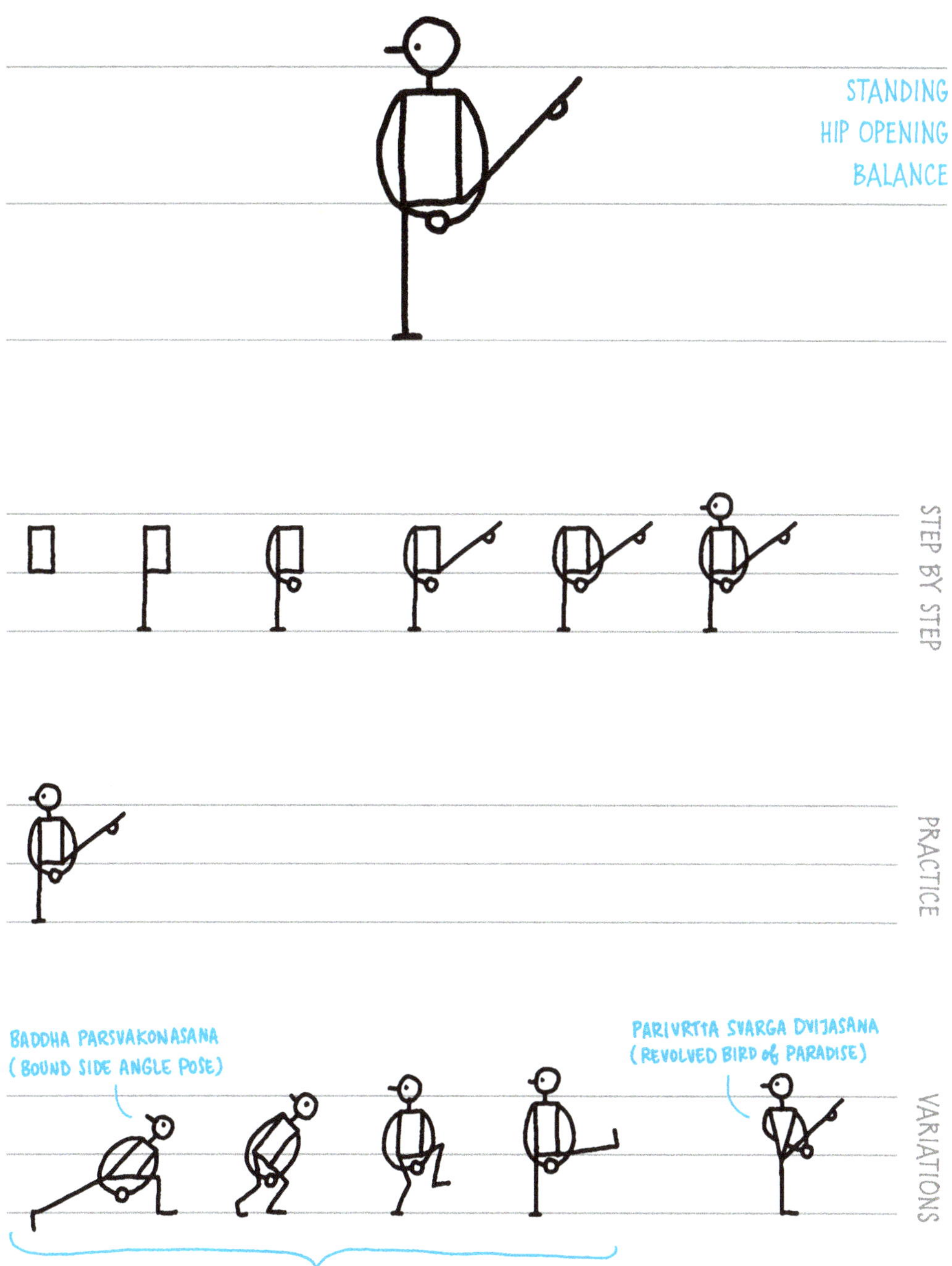

TRIKONASANA

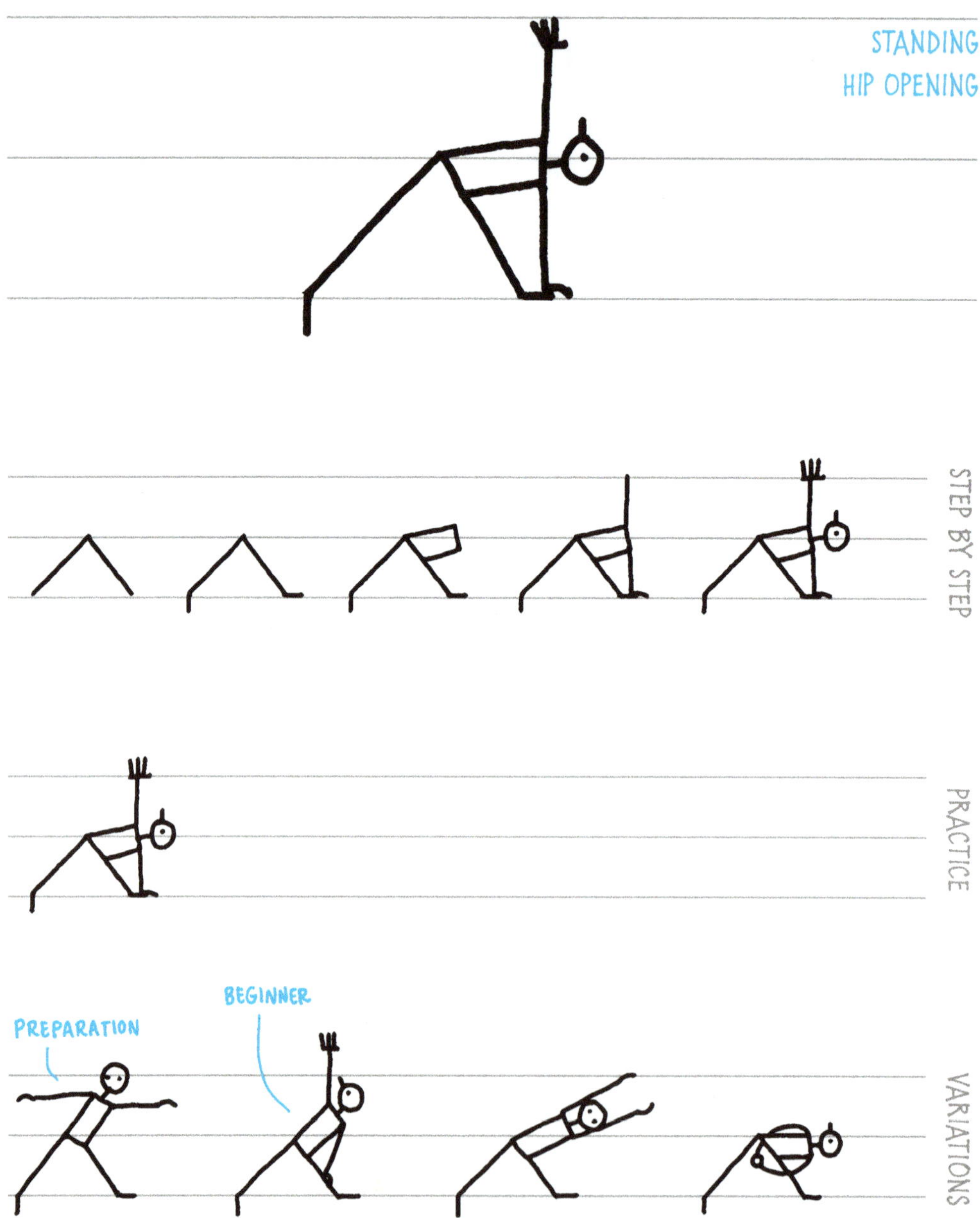

PARIVRTTA TRIKONASANA
REVOLVED TRIANGLE POSE

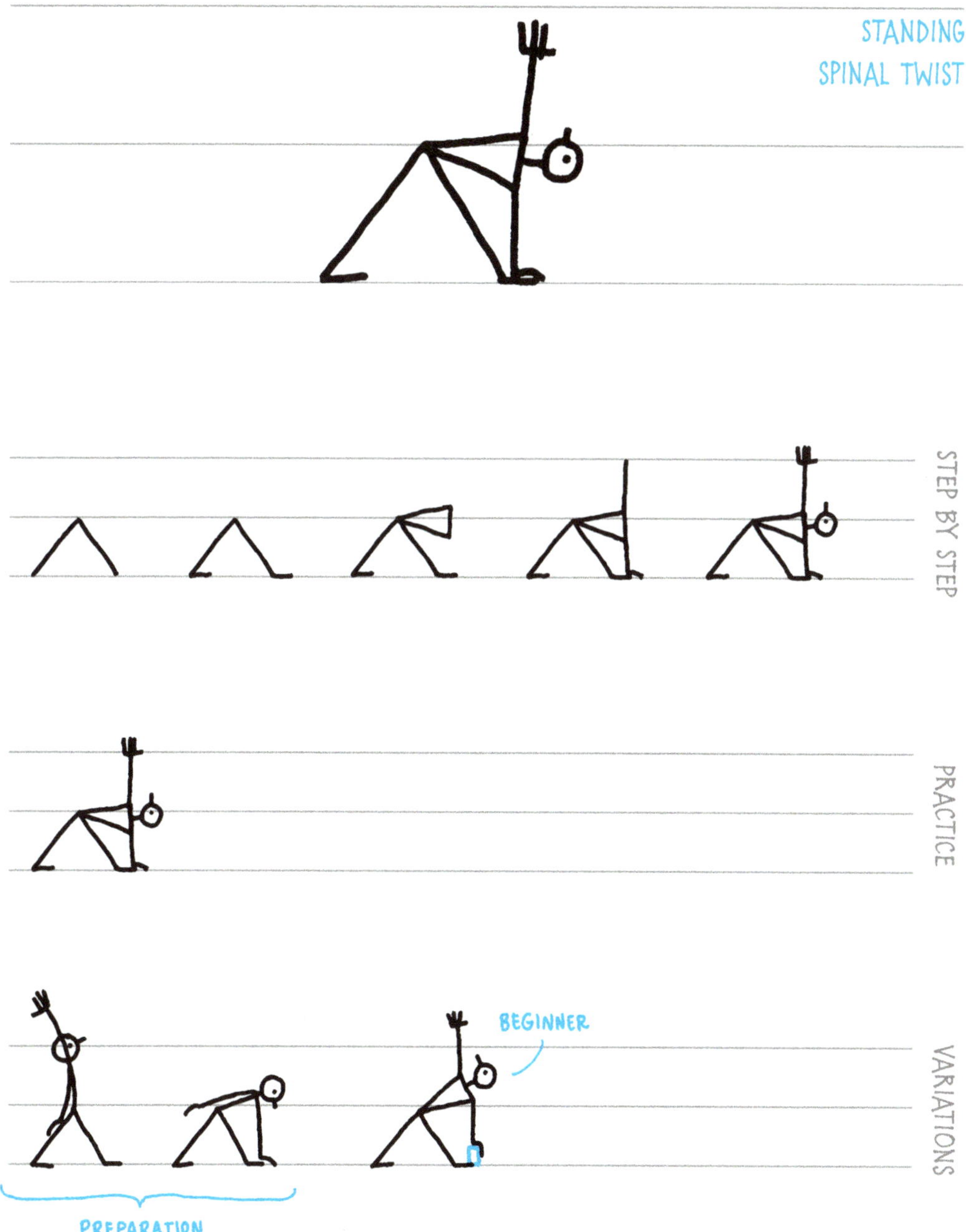

PRASARITA PADOTTANASANA

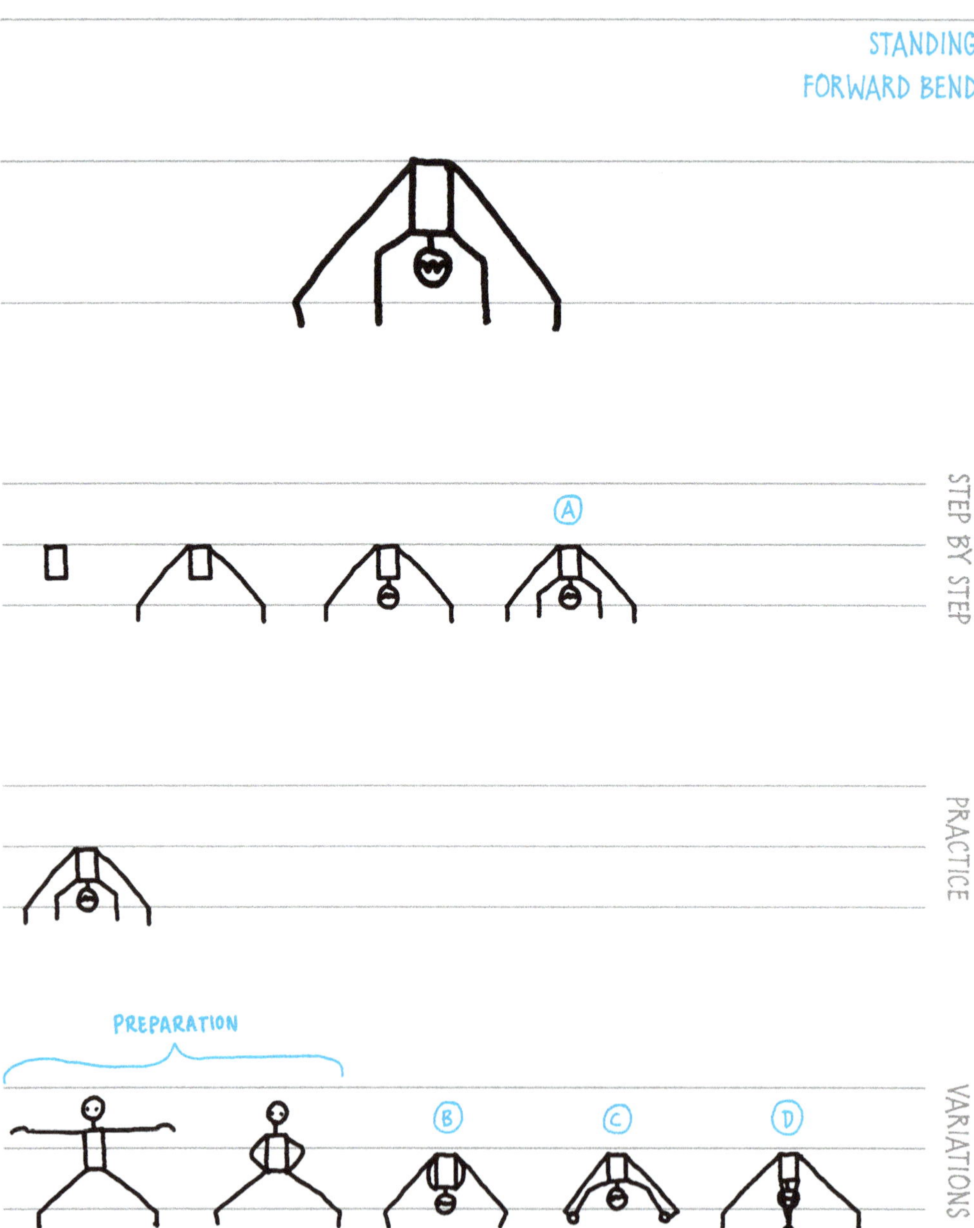

PARSVOTTANASANA

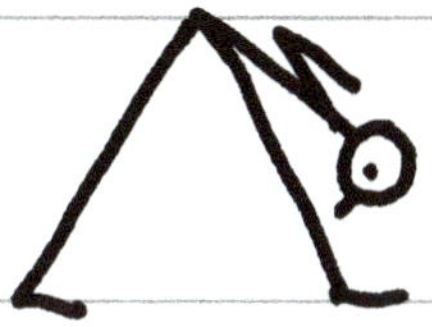

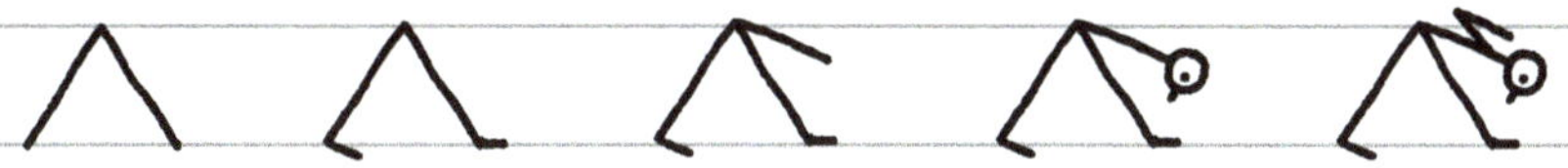

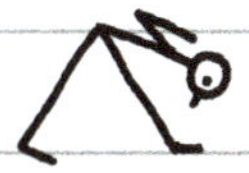

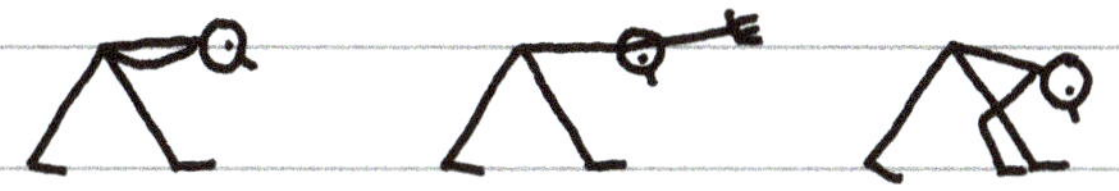

ARDHA CHANDRASANA

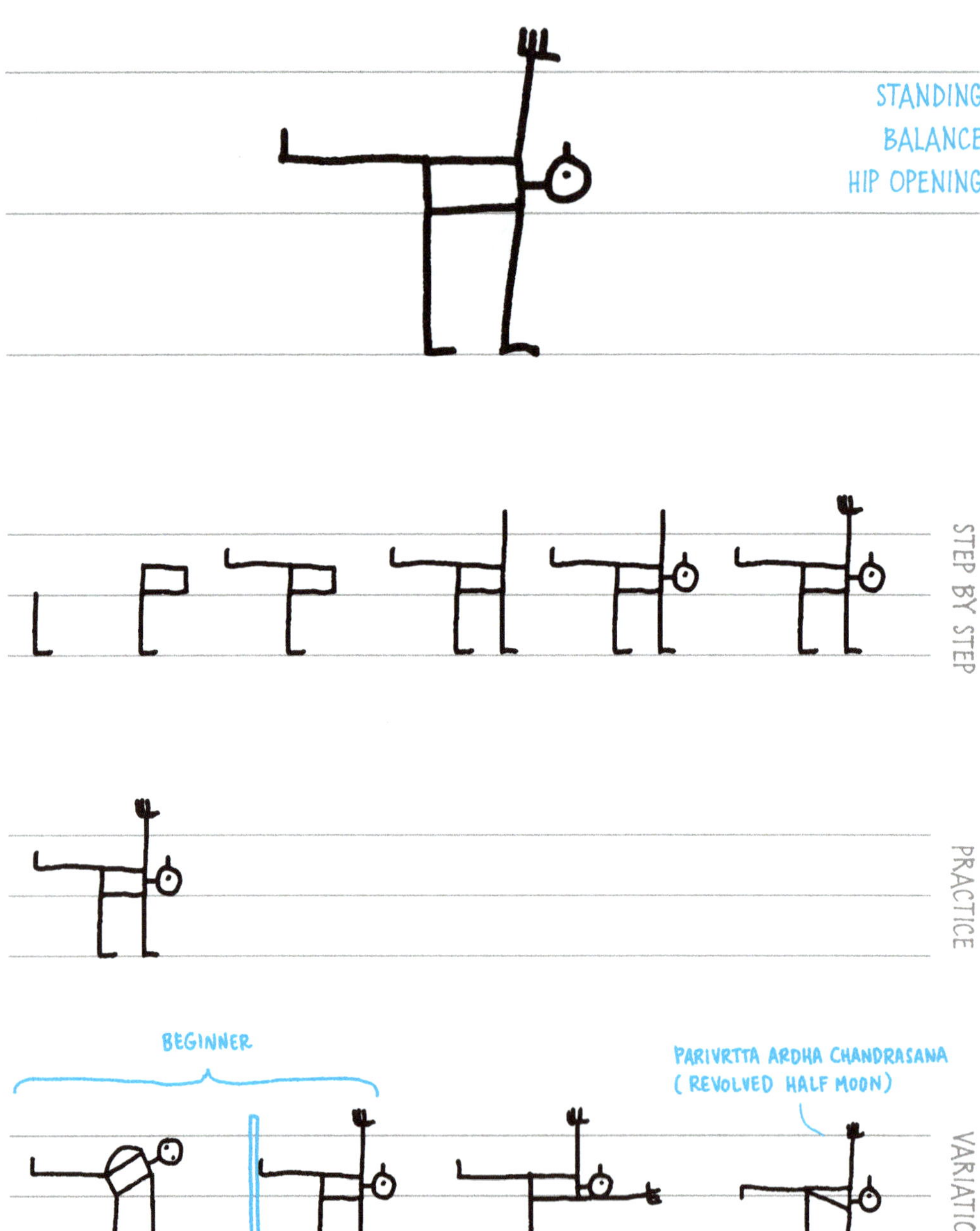

URDHVA PRASARITA EKA PADASANA

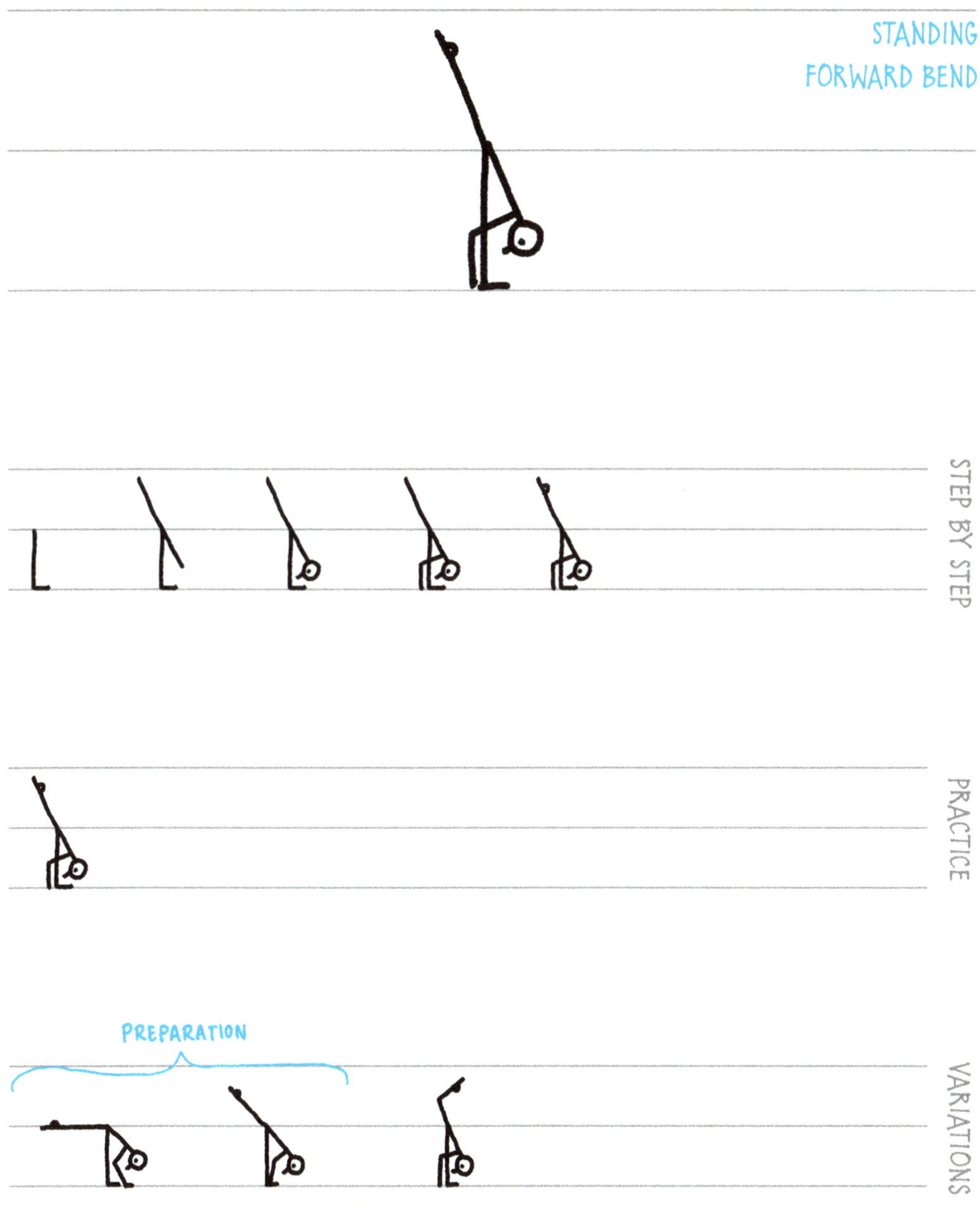

UTKATASANA
CHAIR POSE

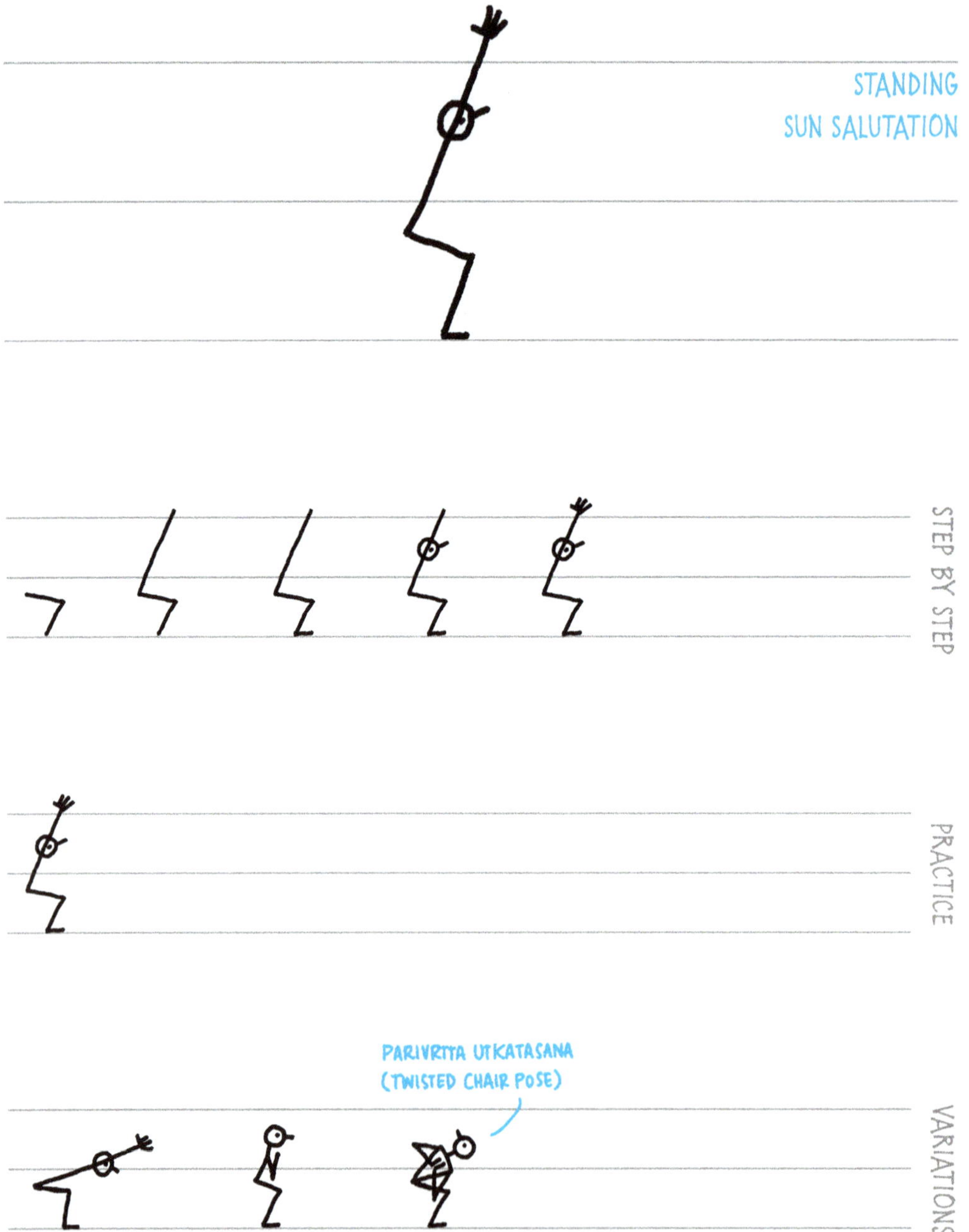

UTKATA KONASANA

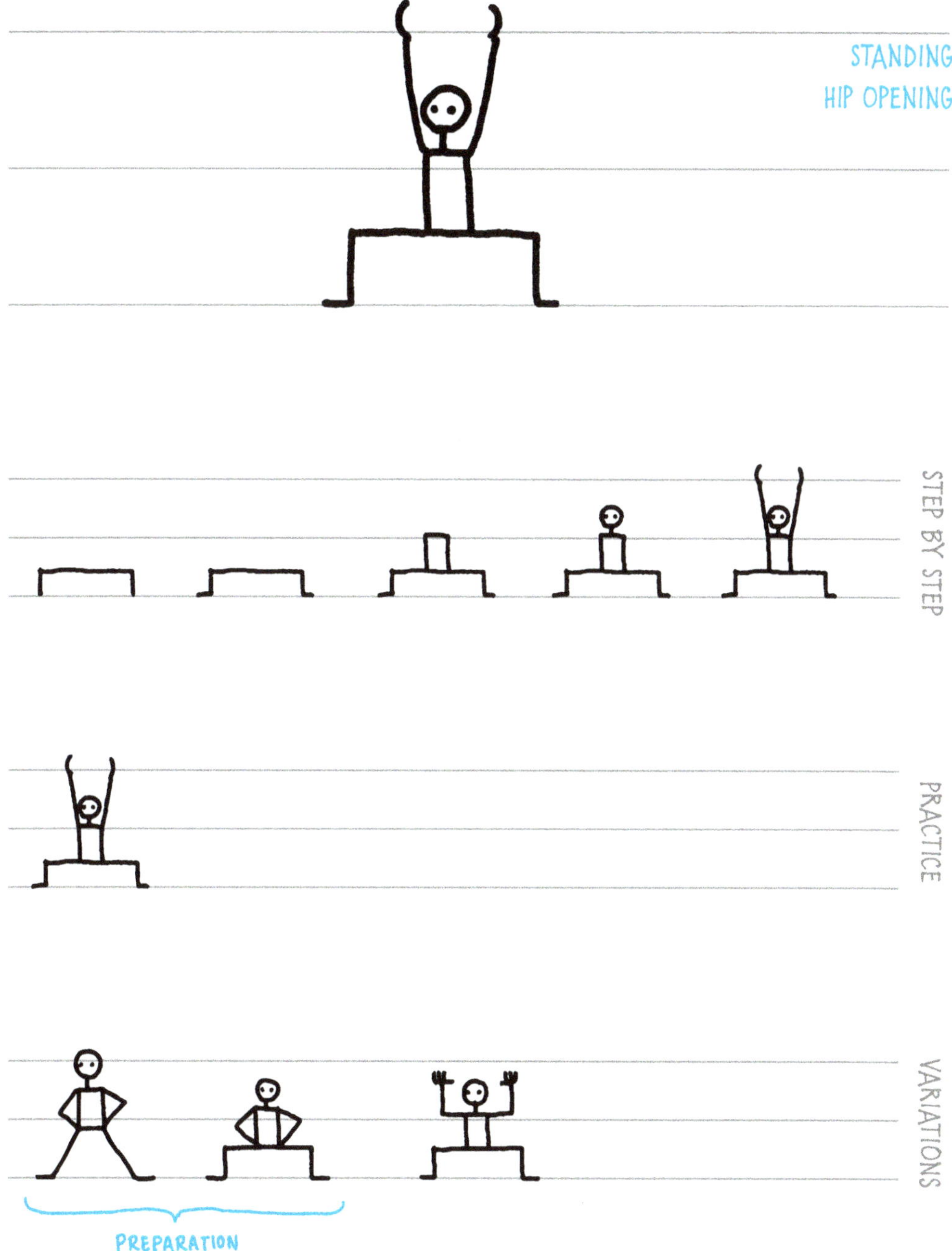

UTTHITA HASTA PADANGUSTASANA

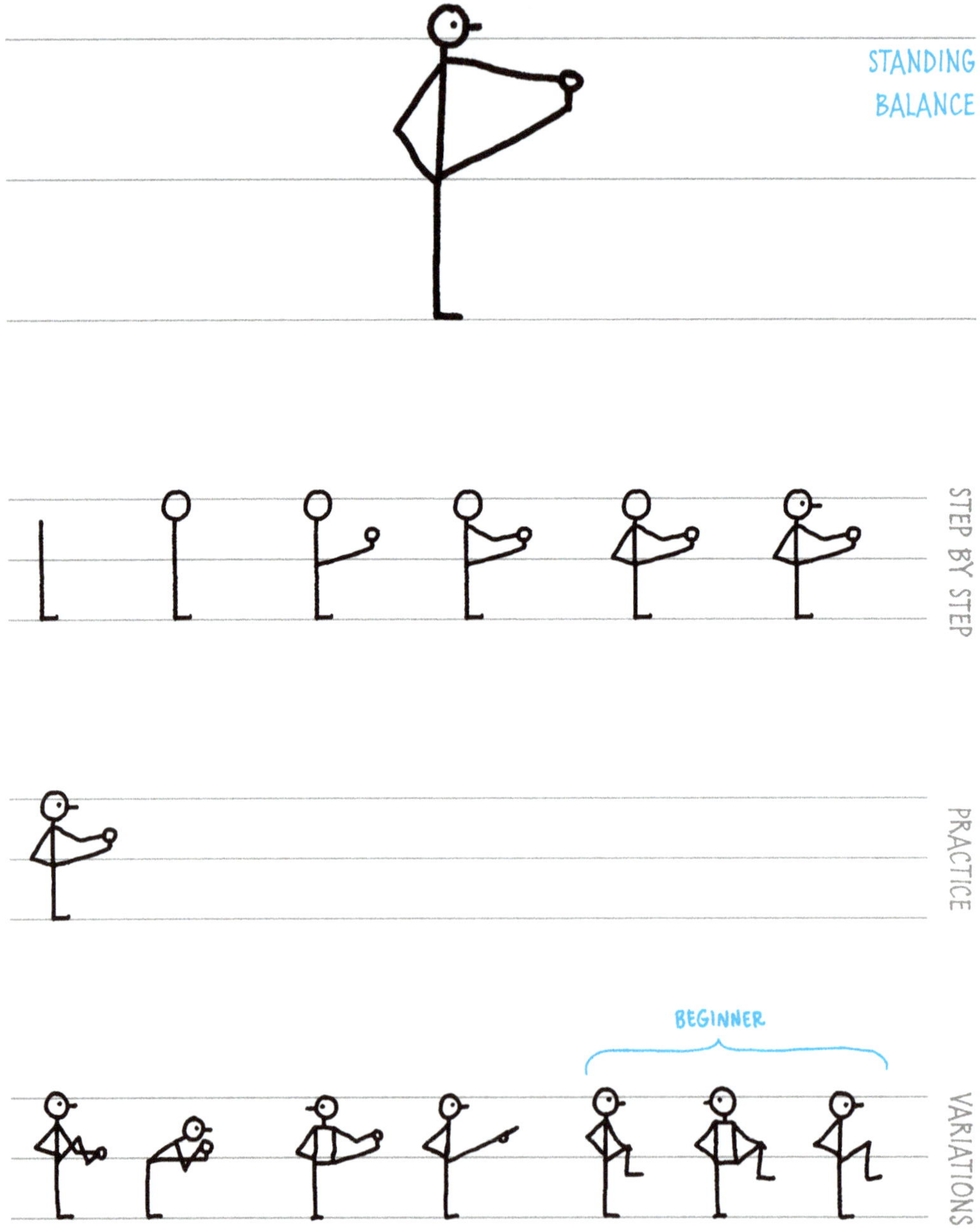

VRKSASANA

TREE POSE

STANDING
BALANCE
STEP BY STEP
PRACTICE
ARDHA BADDHA PADMOTTANASANA
(HALF BOUND FORWARD FOLD)
VARIATIONS

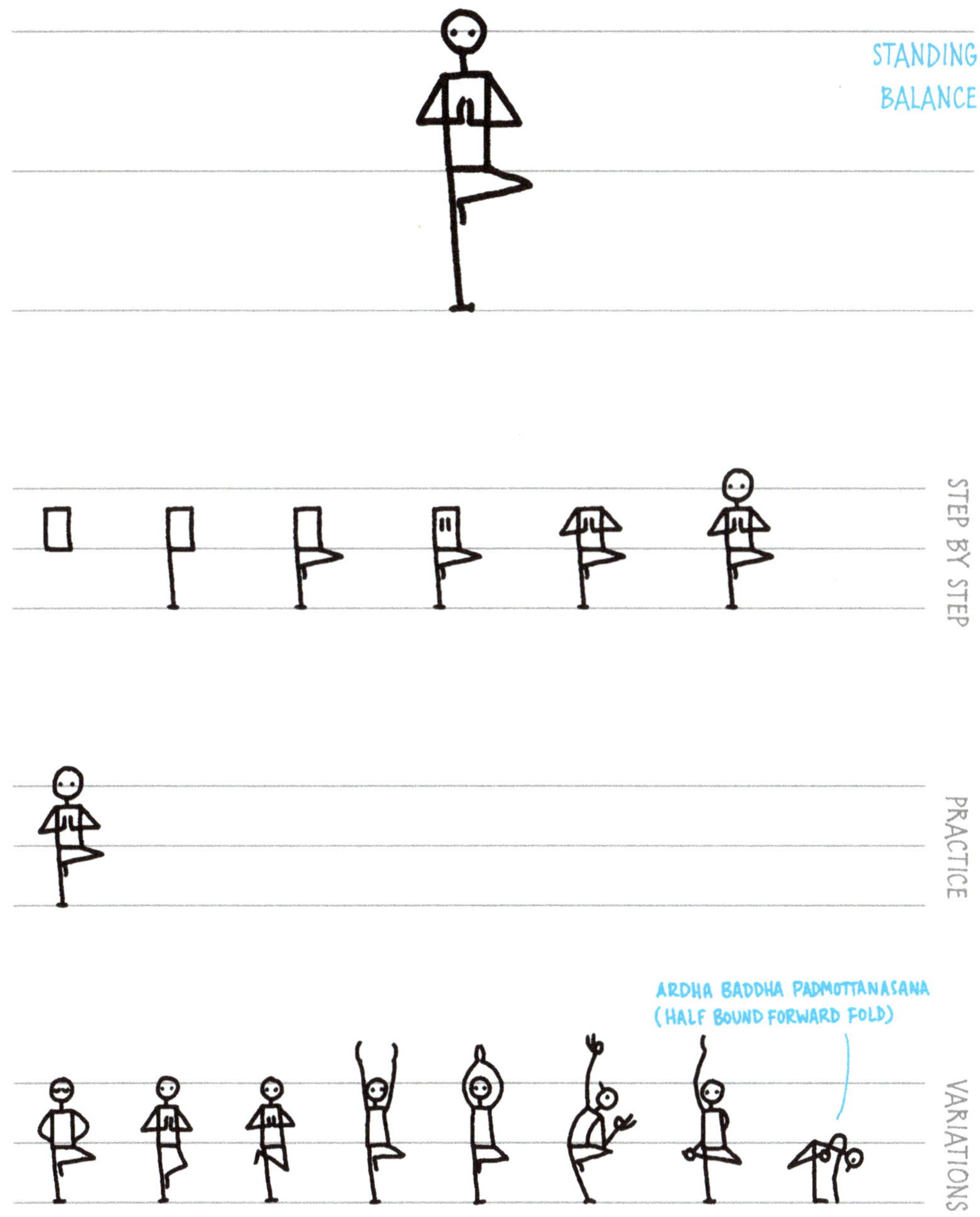

NATARAJASANA

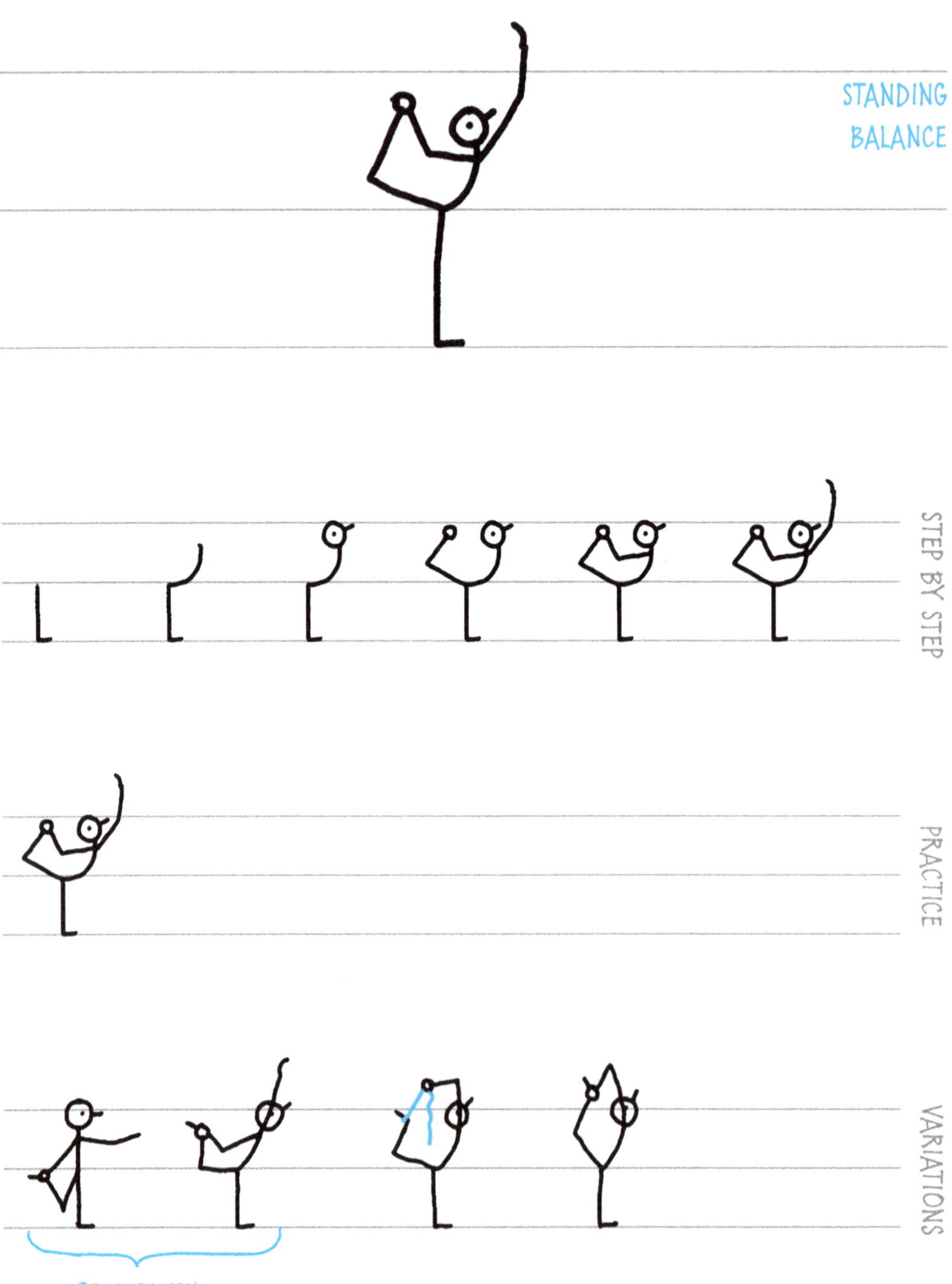

GARUDASANA
EAGLE POSE

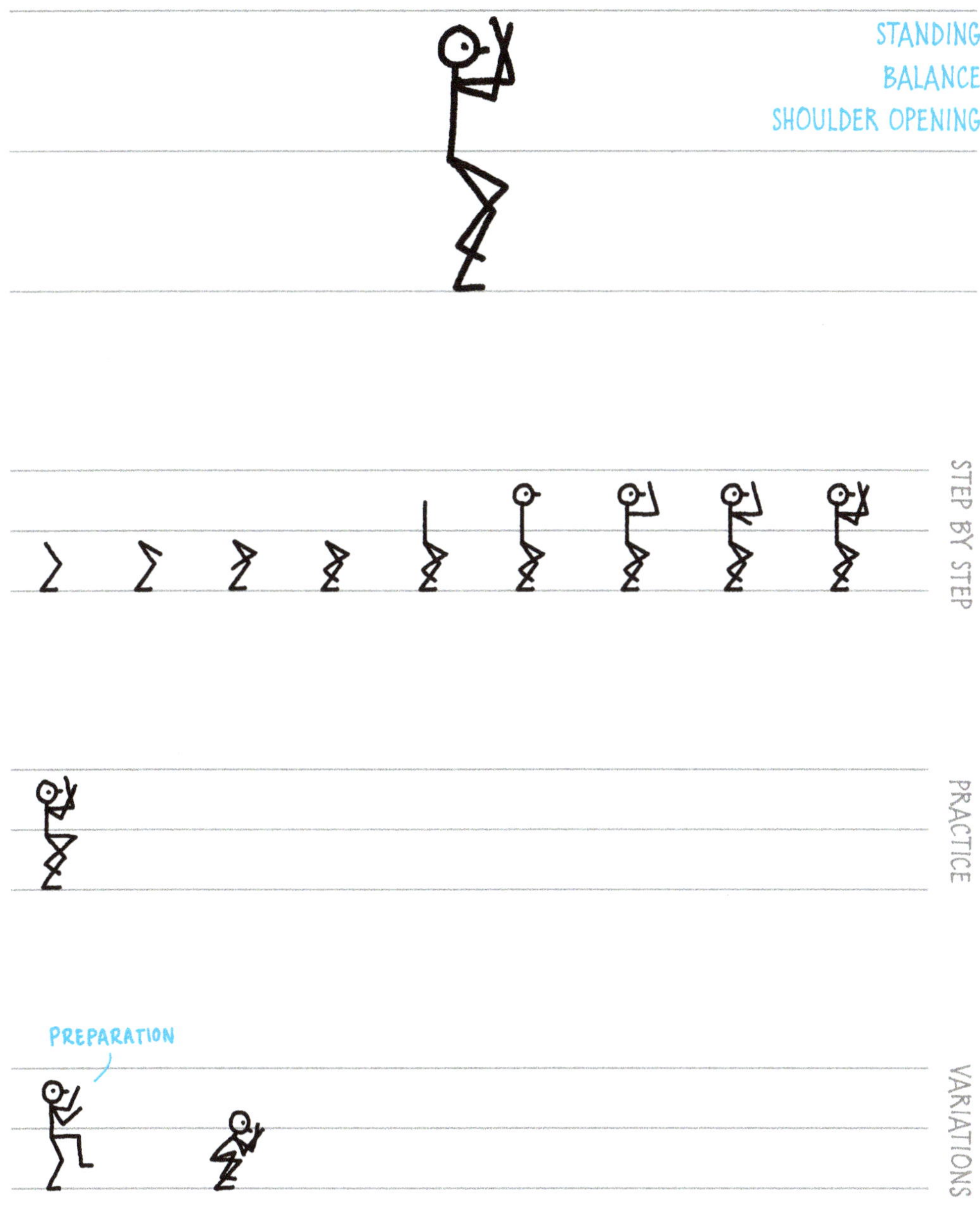

MALASANA
GARLAND POSE

STANDING
HIP OPENING

STEP BY STEP

PRACTICE

PASASANA
(NOOSE POSE)

VARIATIONS

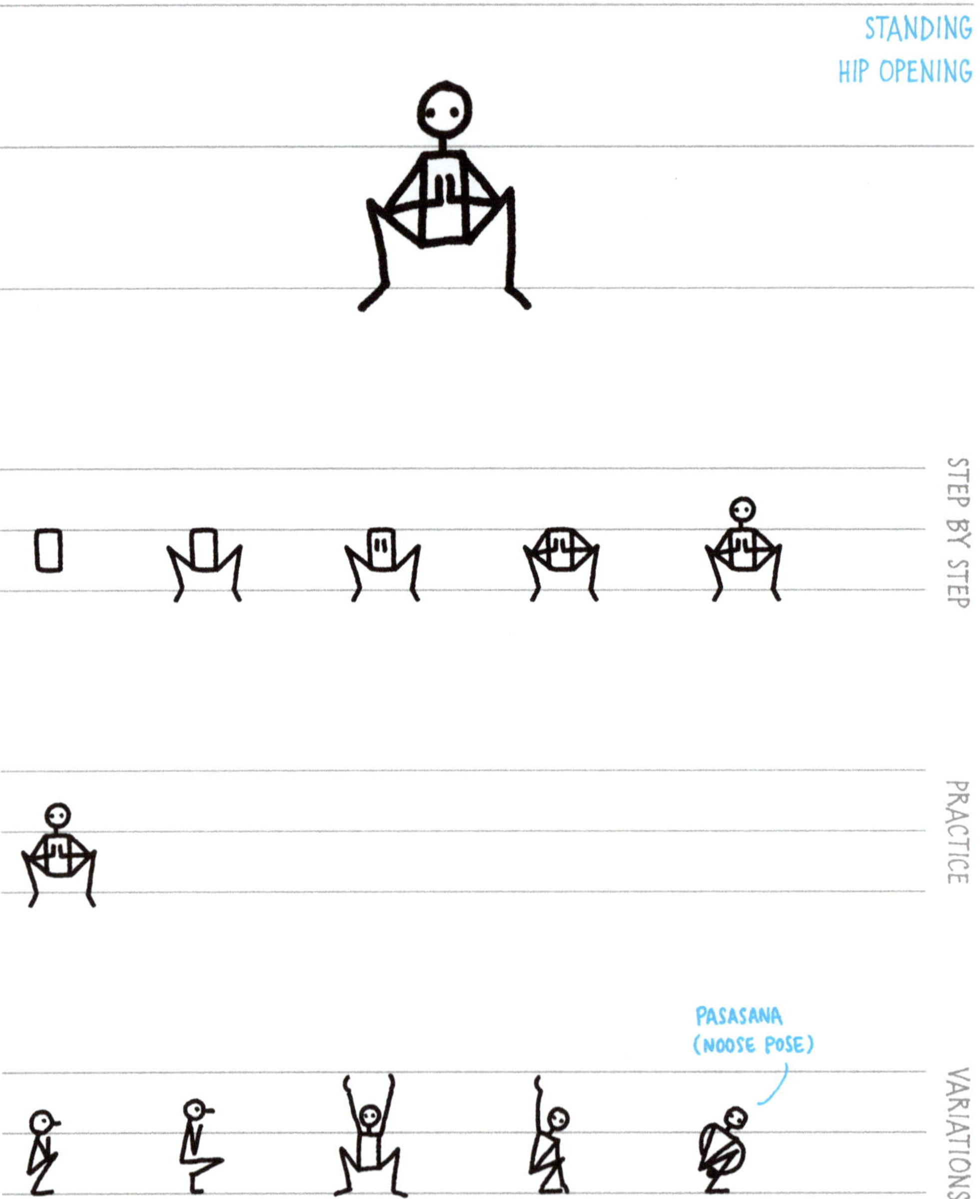

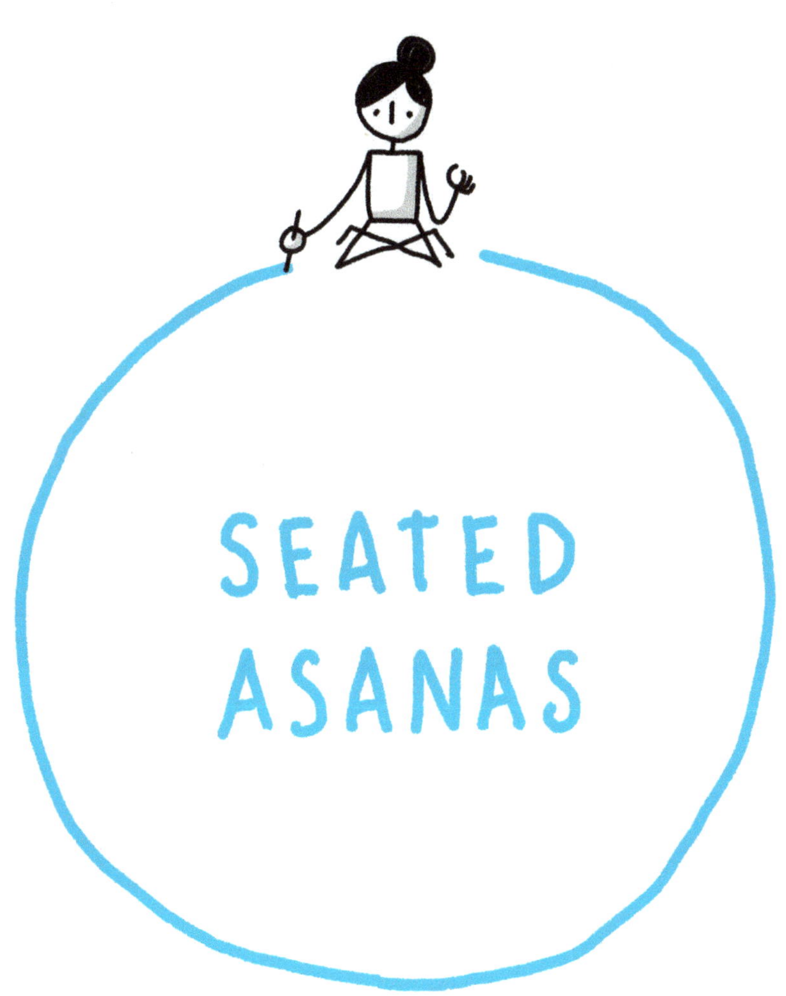

SEATED ASANAS

PADMASANA
LOTUS POSE

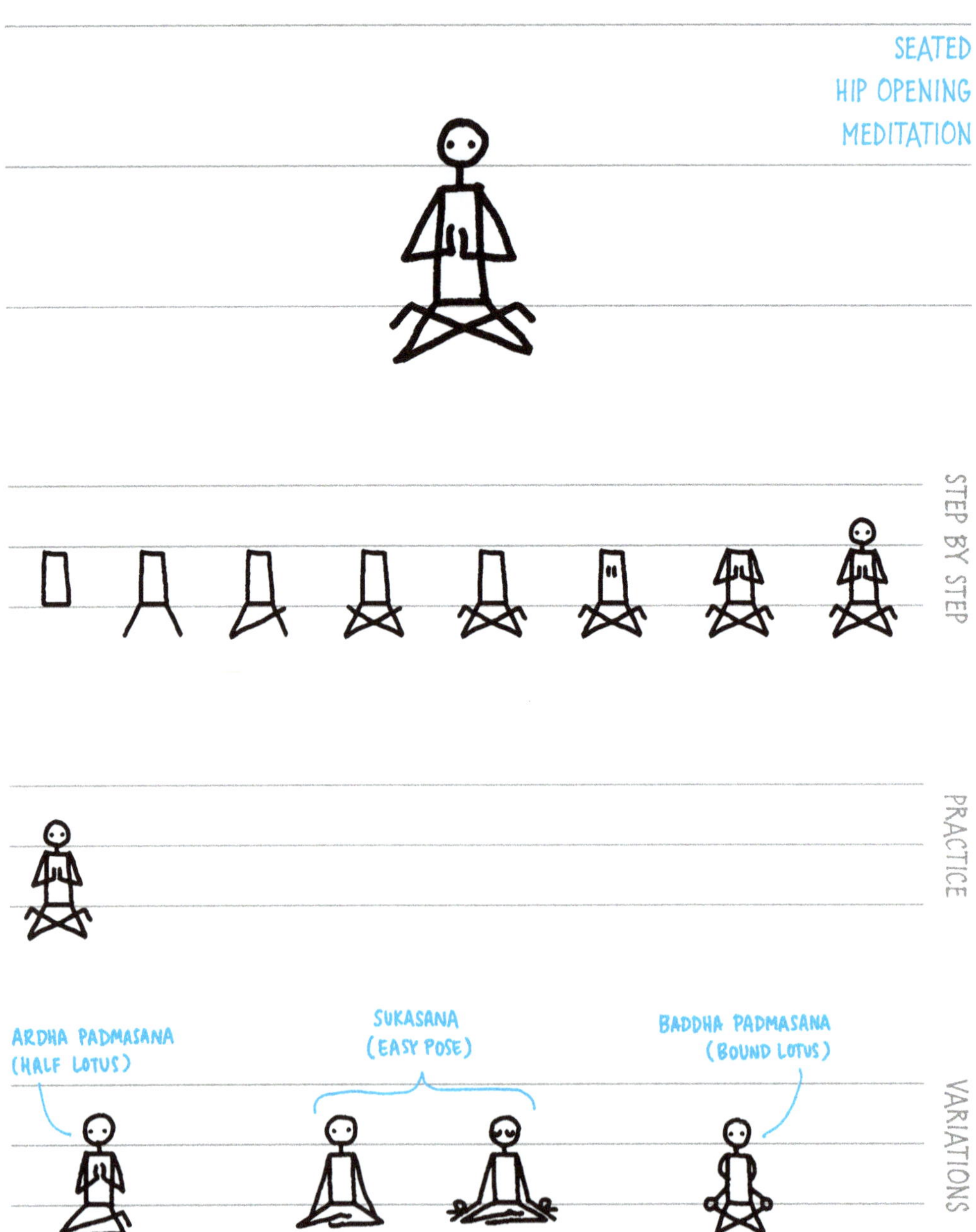

DANDASANA

STAFF POSE

SEATED
STEP BY STEP
PRACTICE
BEGINNER
VARIATIONS

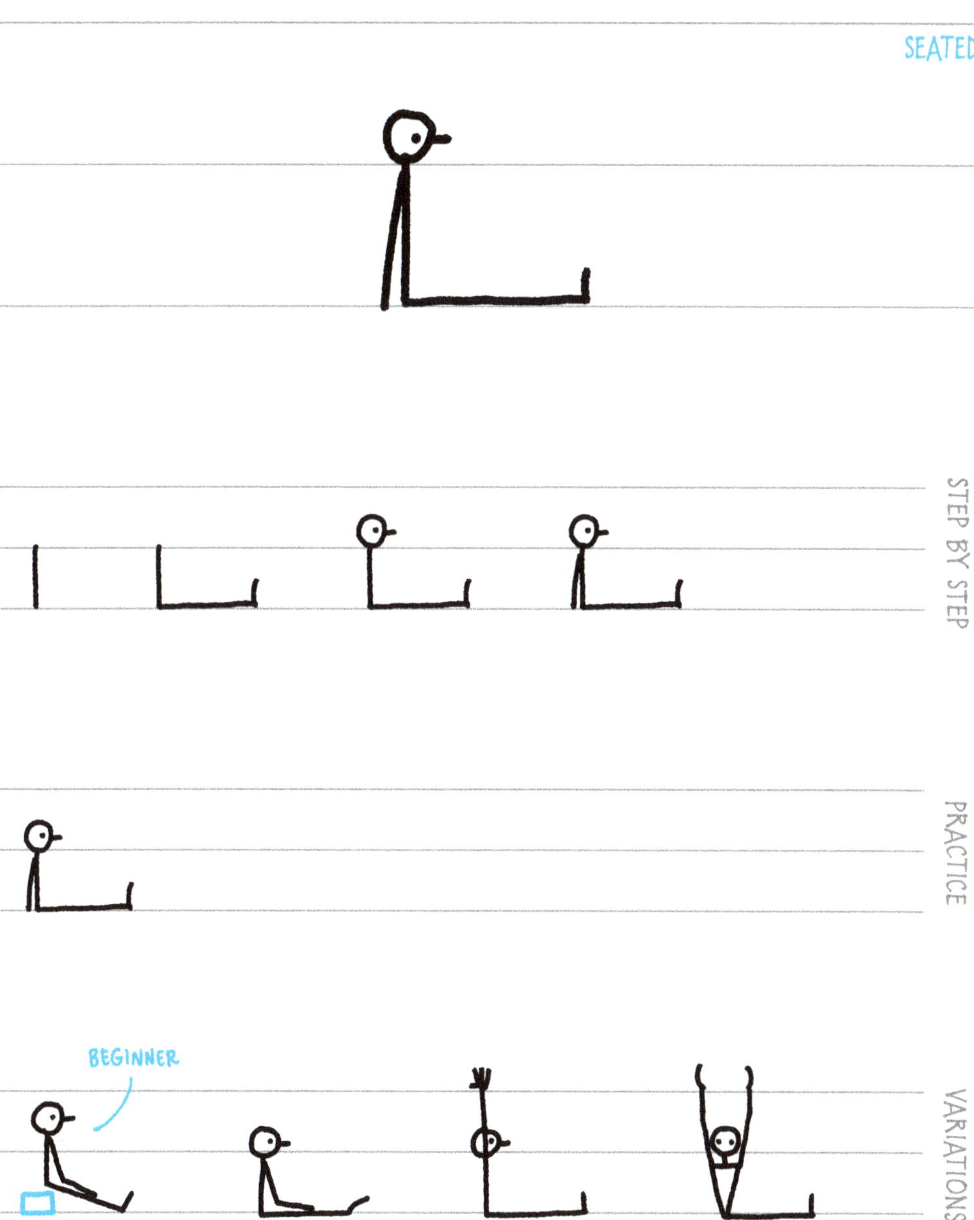

PASCHIMOTTANASANA

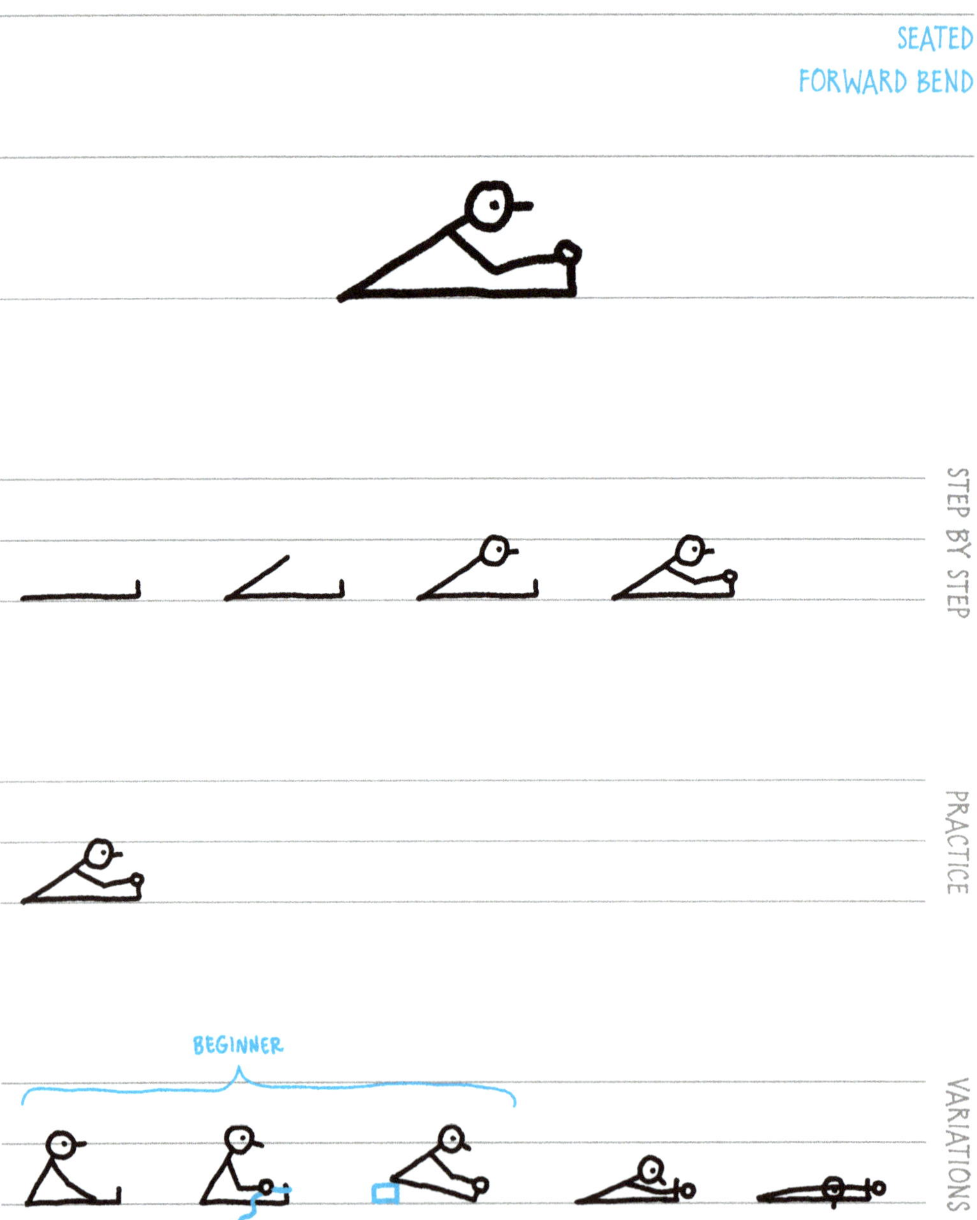

JANU SIRSASANA

HEAD-TO-KNEE POSE

SEATED
FORWARD BEND
HIP OPENING

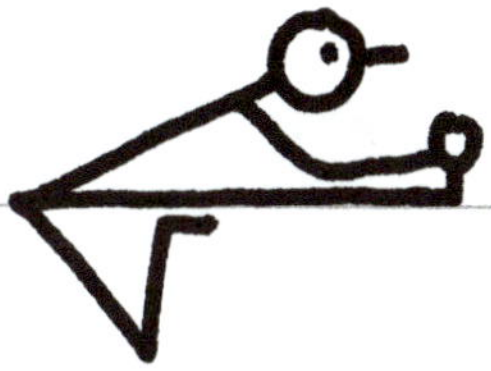

STEP BY STEP

PRACTICE

VARIATIONS

BEGINNER
ARDHA BADDHA PADMA PASCHIMOTTANASANA (INTENSE FORWARD FOLD WITH BOUND HALF LOTUS)

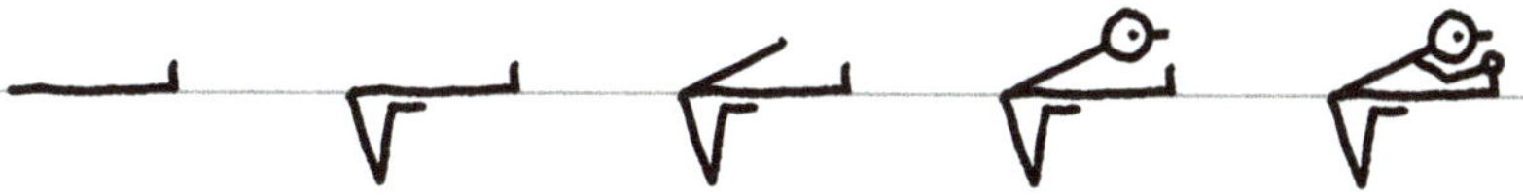

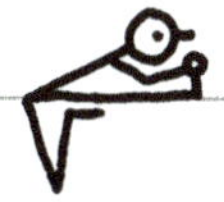

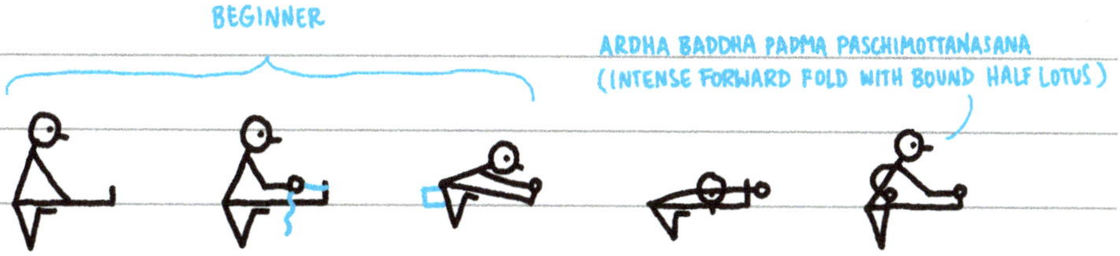

PARIVRTTA JANU SIRSASANA

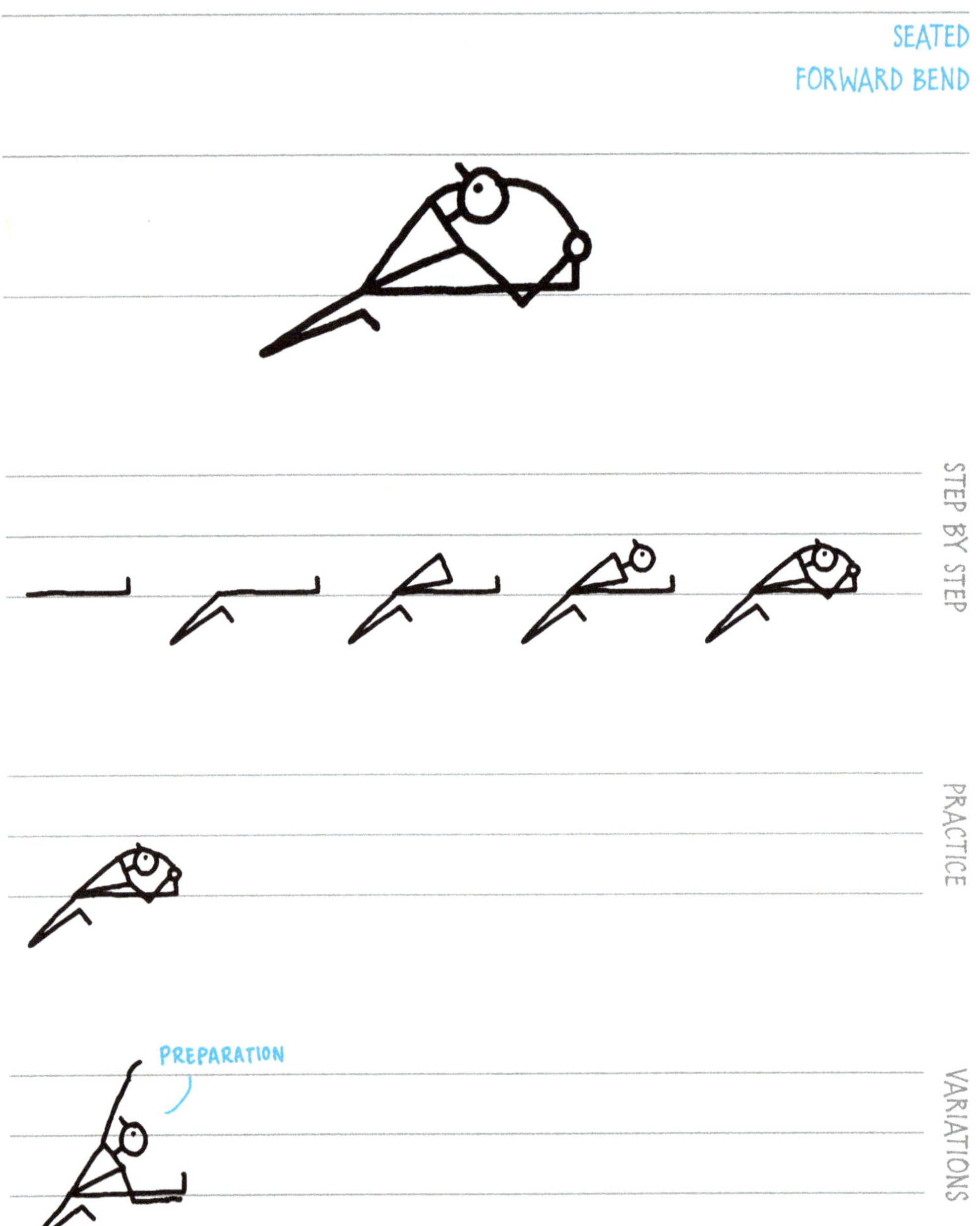

UPAVISTHA KONASANA
WIDE-ANGLE SEATED FORWARD FOLD

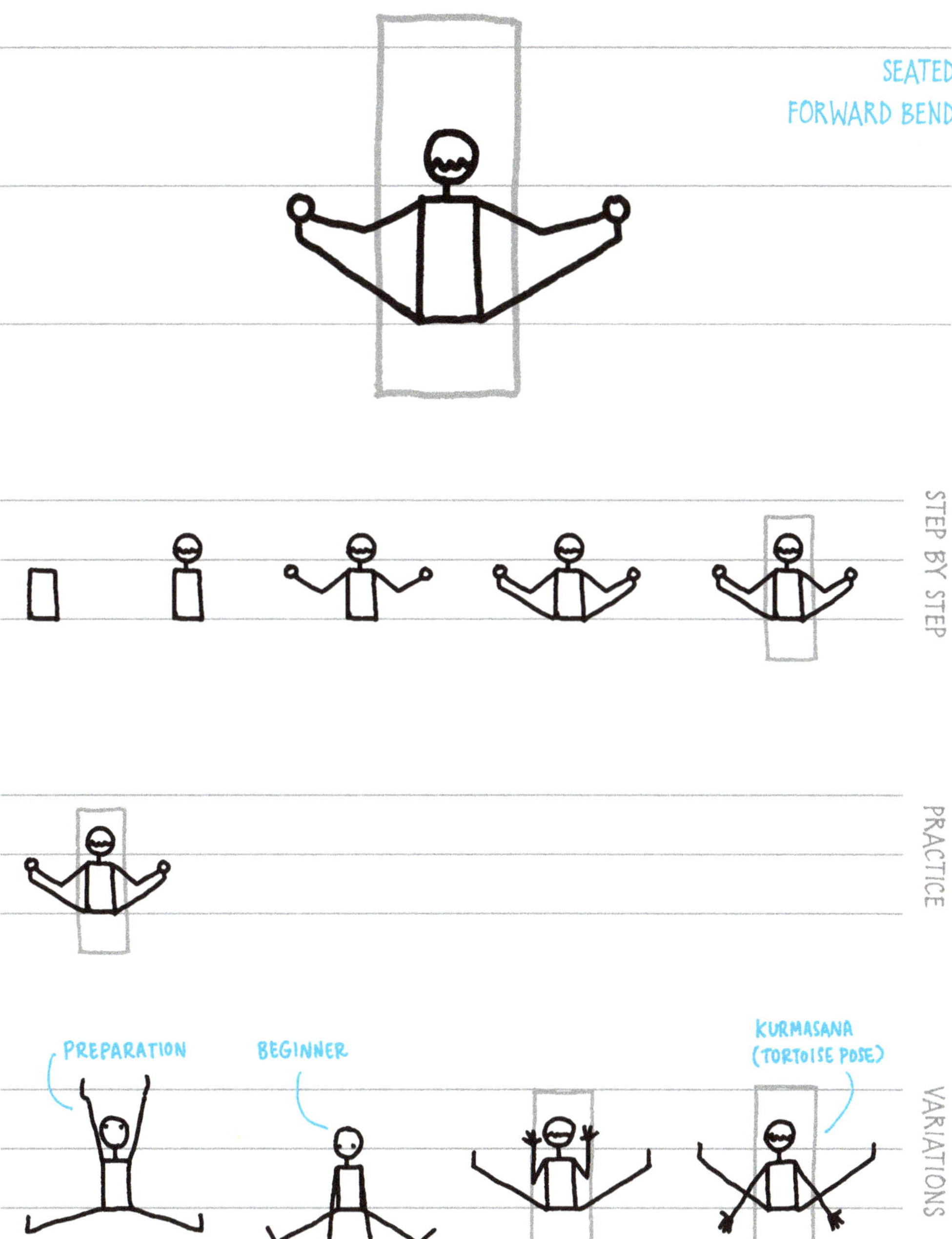

MARICHIASANA

POSE OF THE SAGE MARICHI

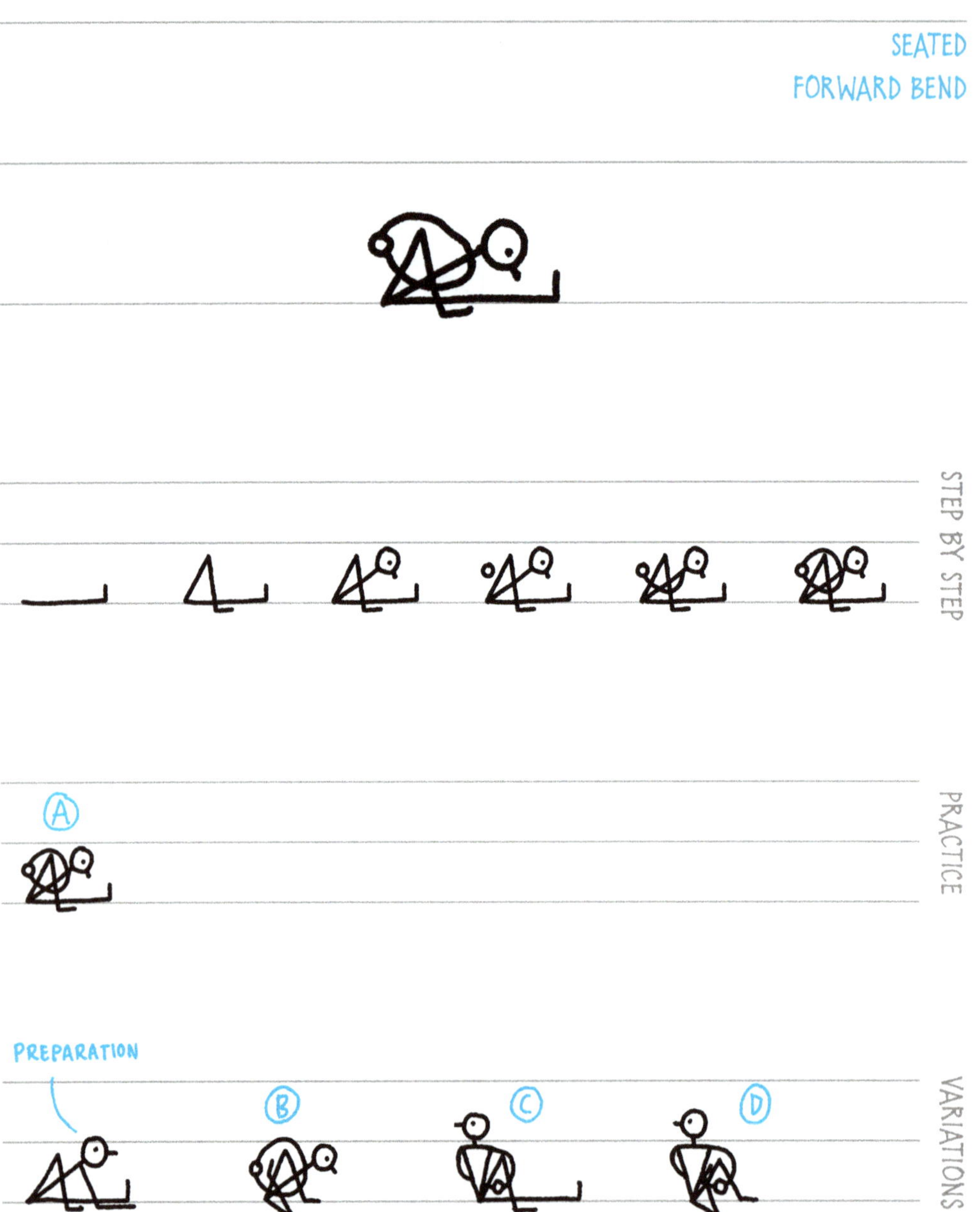

ARDHA MATSYENDRASANA

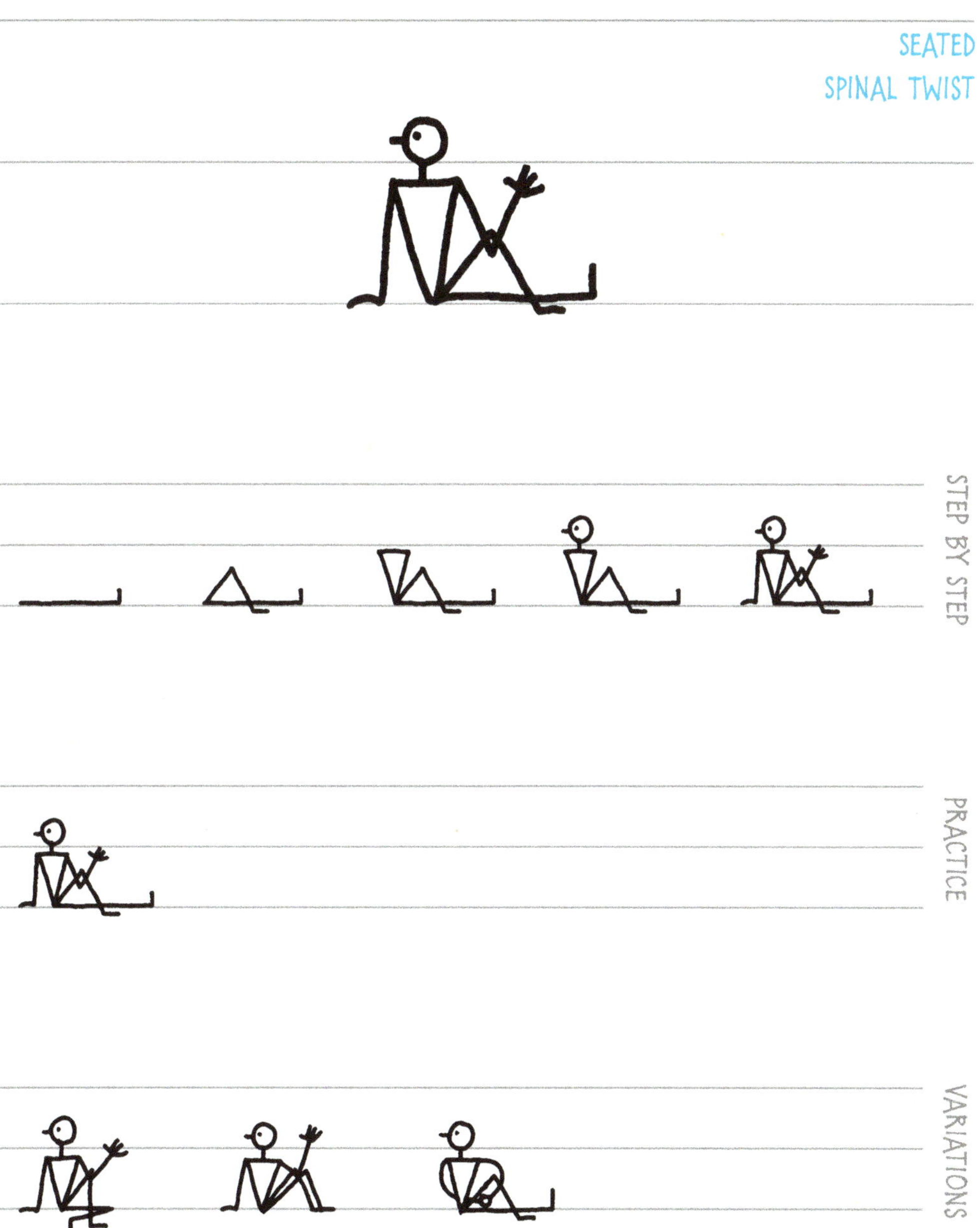

GOMUKHASANA
COW FACE POSE

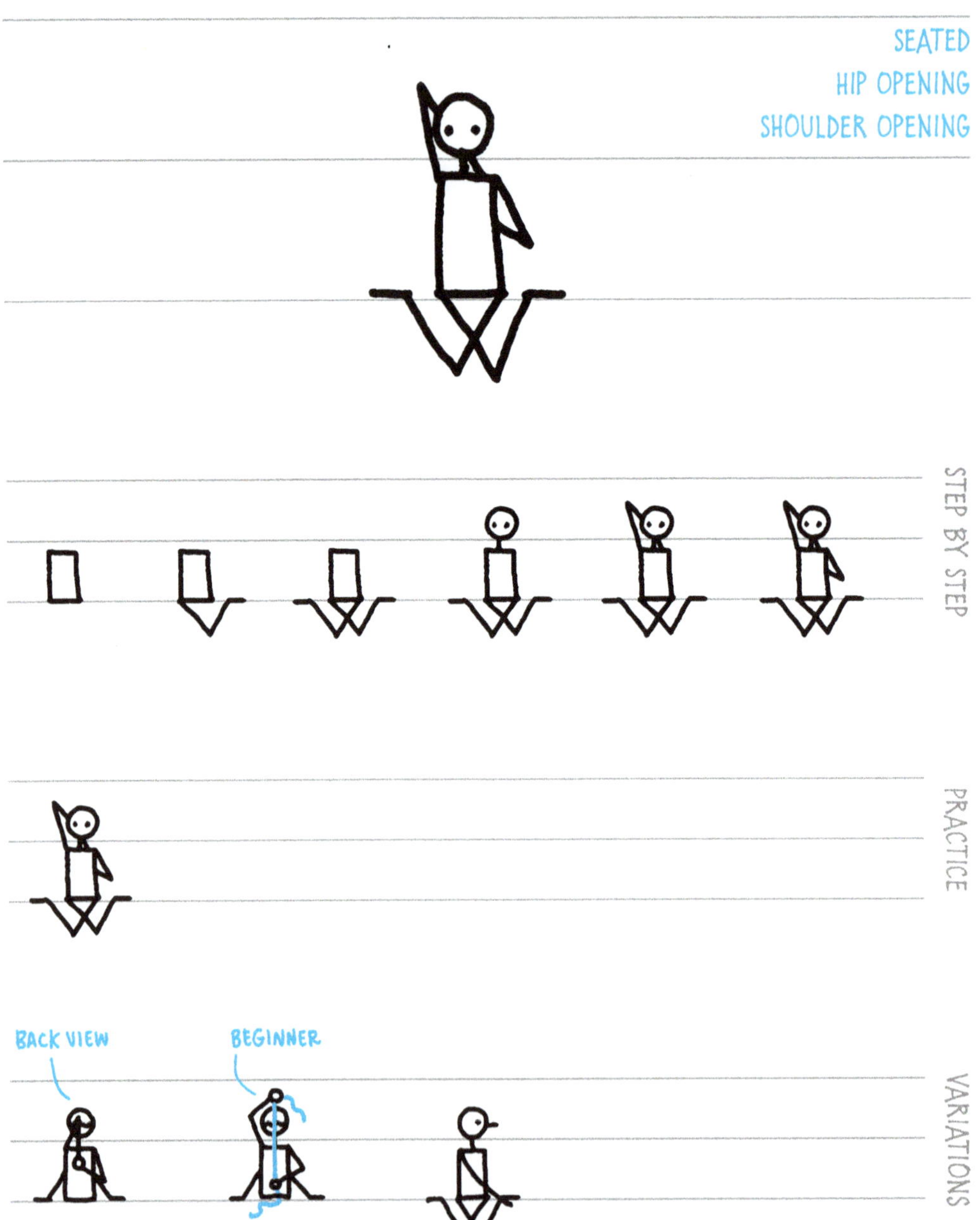

AGNISTAMBHASANA

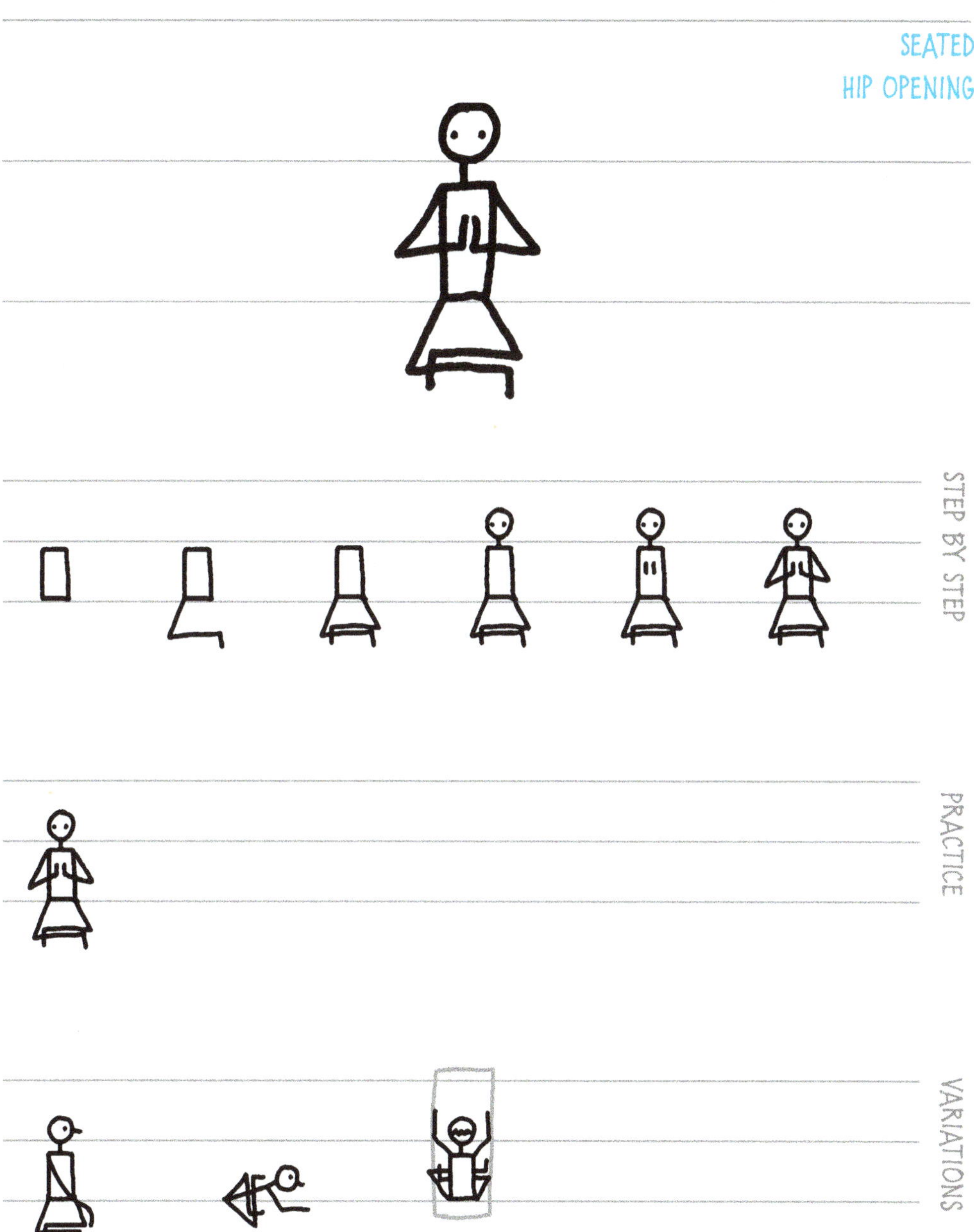

BADDHAKONASANA
BOUND ANGLE POSE

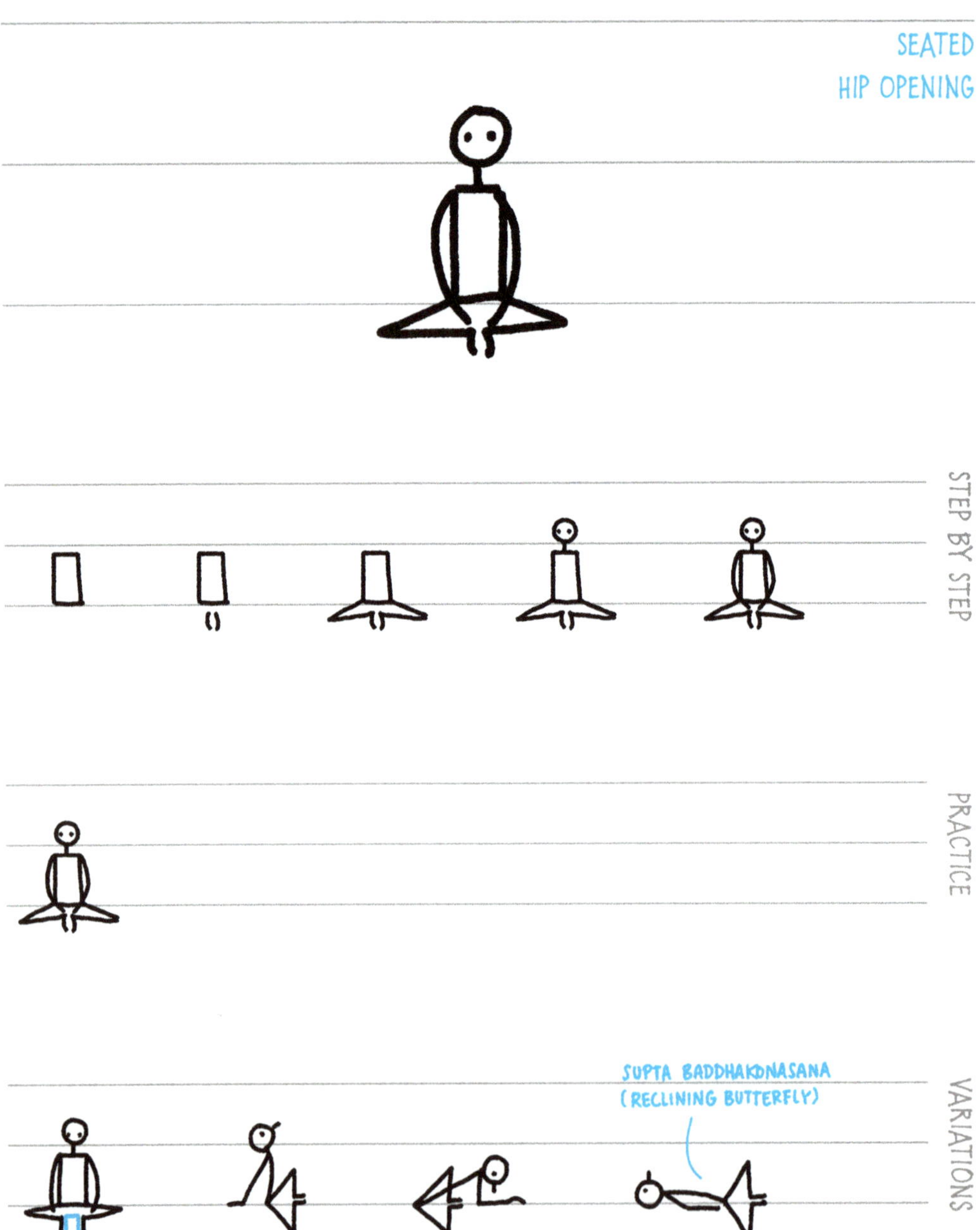

NAVASANA
BOAT POSE

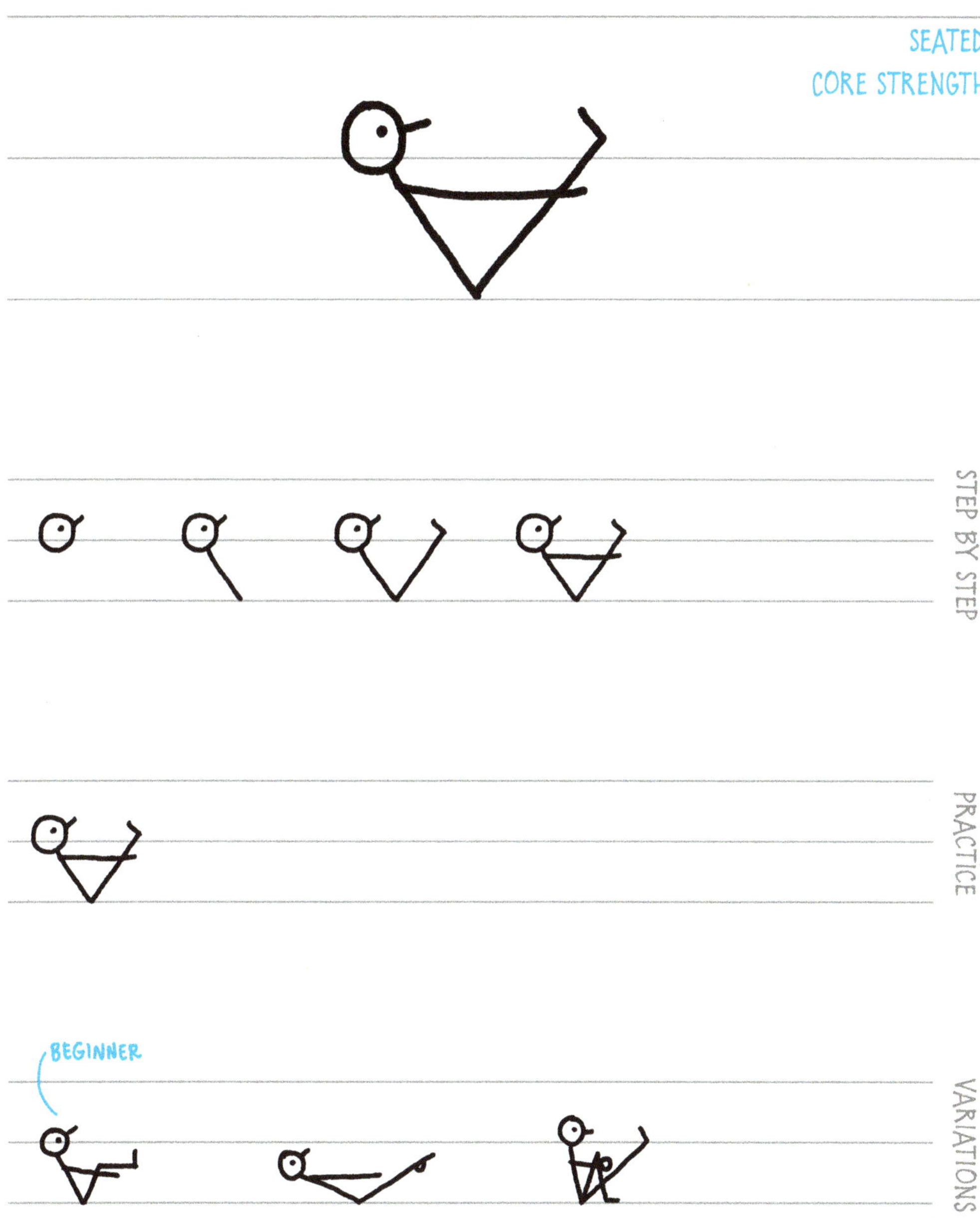

HANUMANASANA

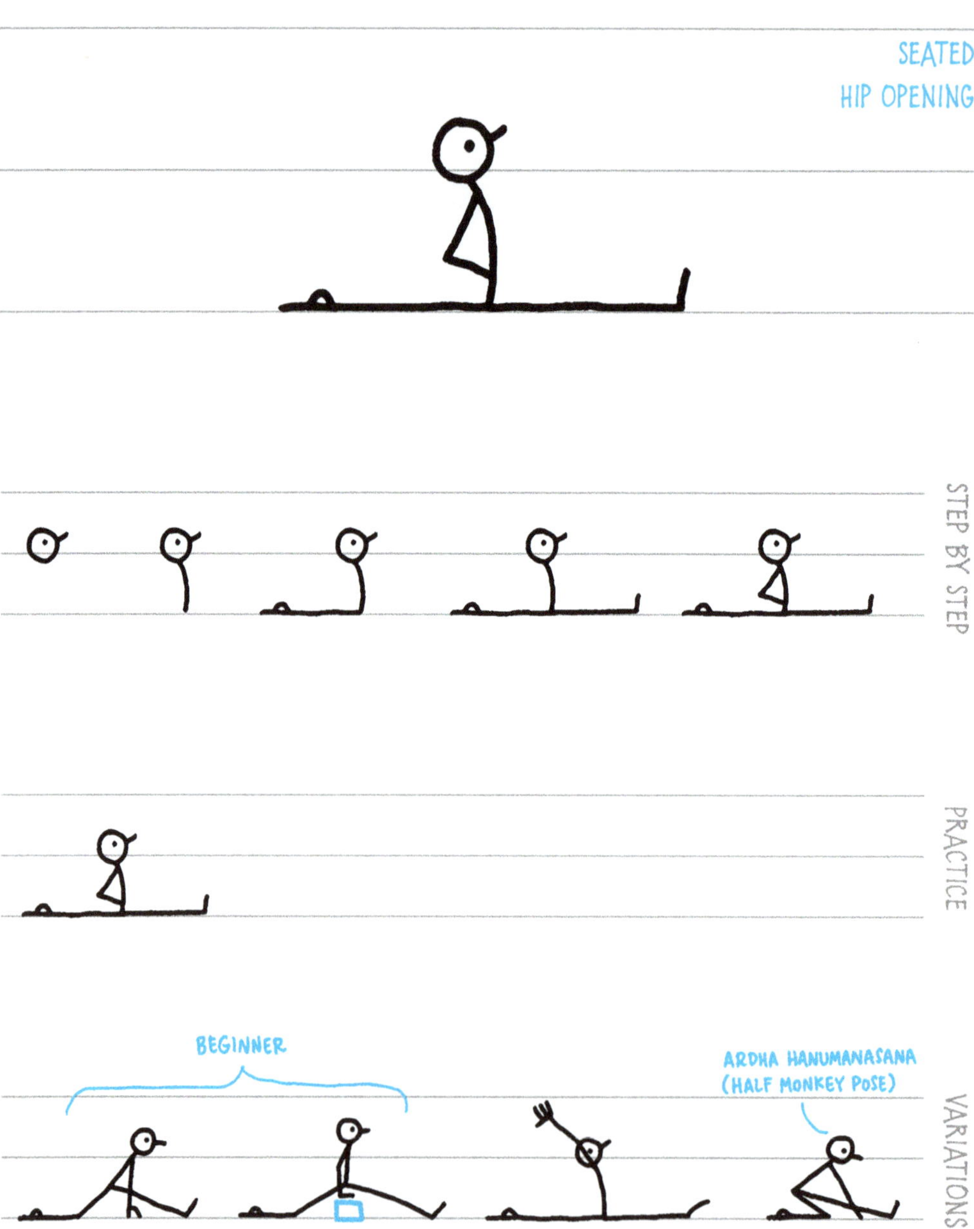

KAPOTASANA
PIGEON POSE

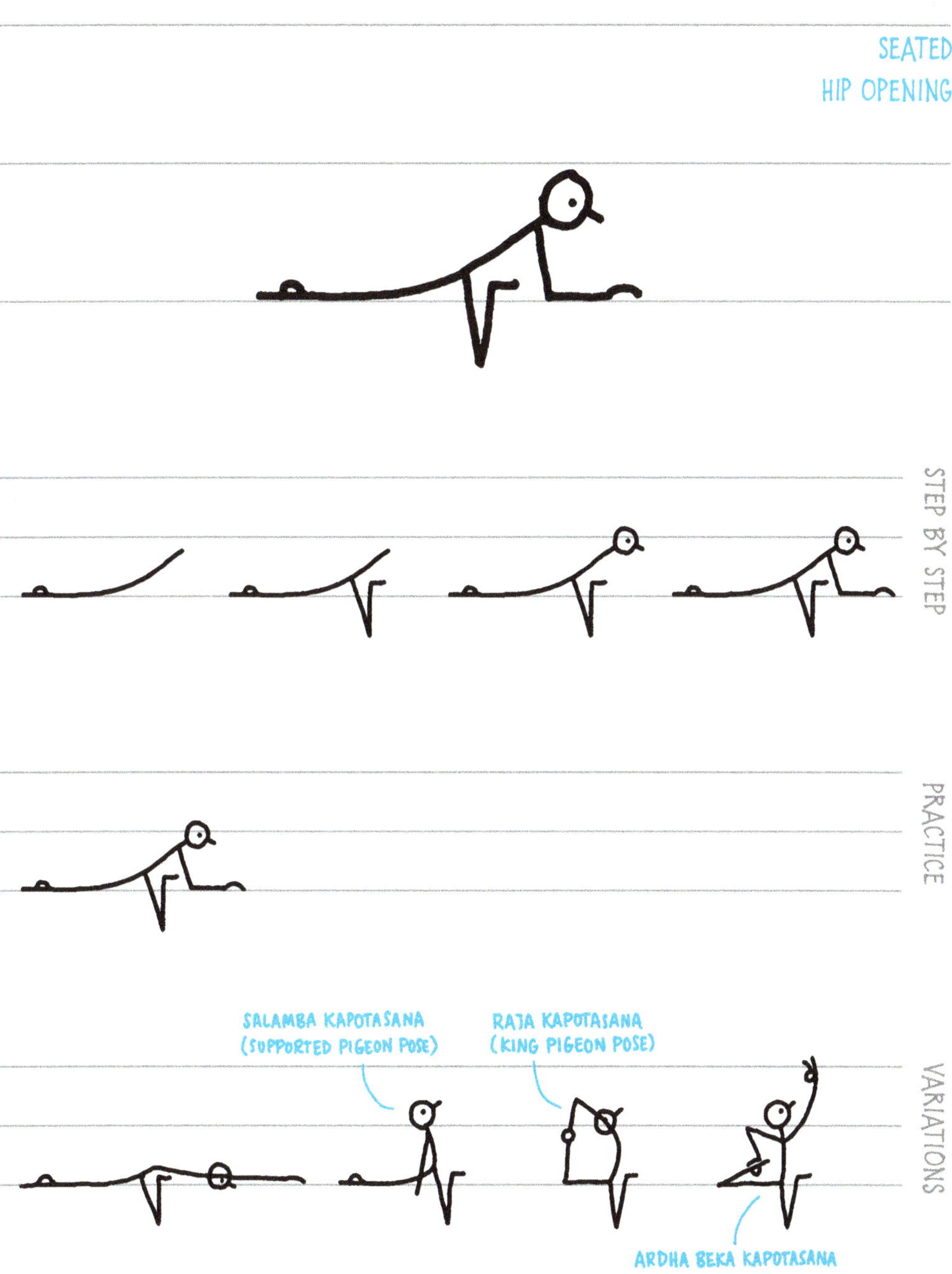

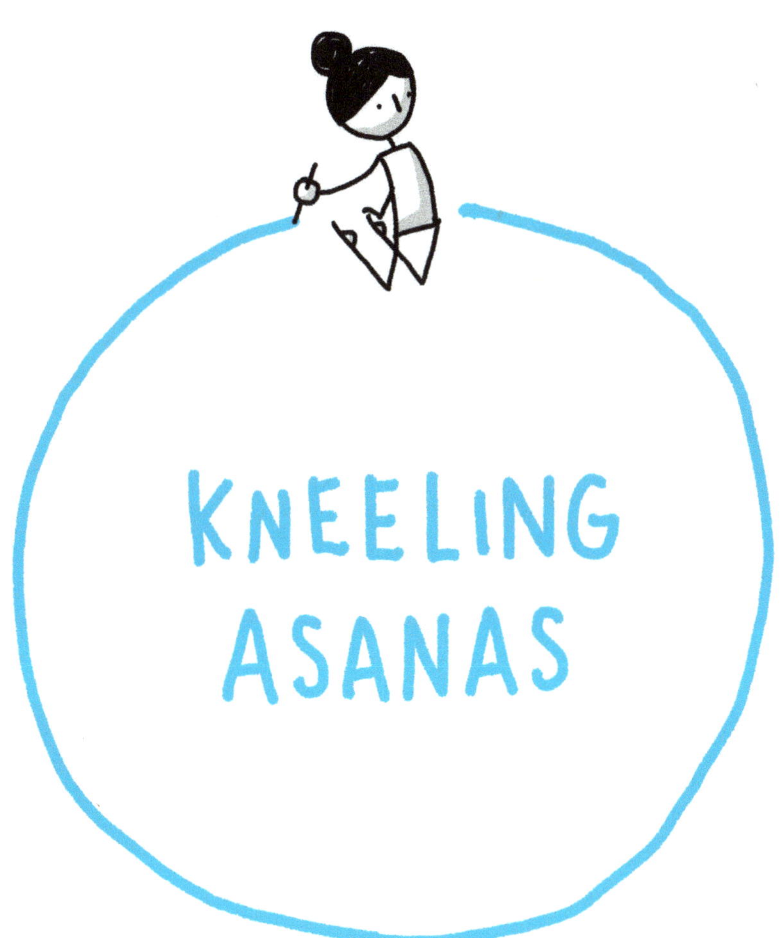

KNEELING ASANAS

VAJRASANA
THUNDERBOLT POSE

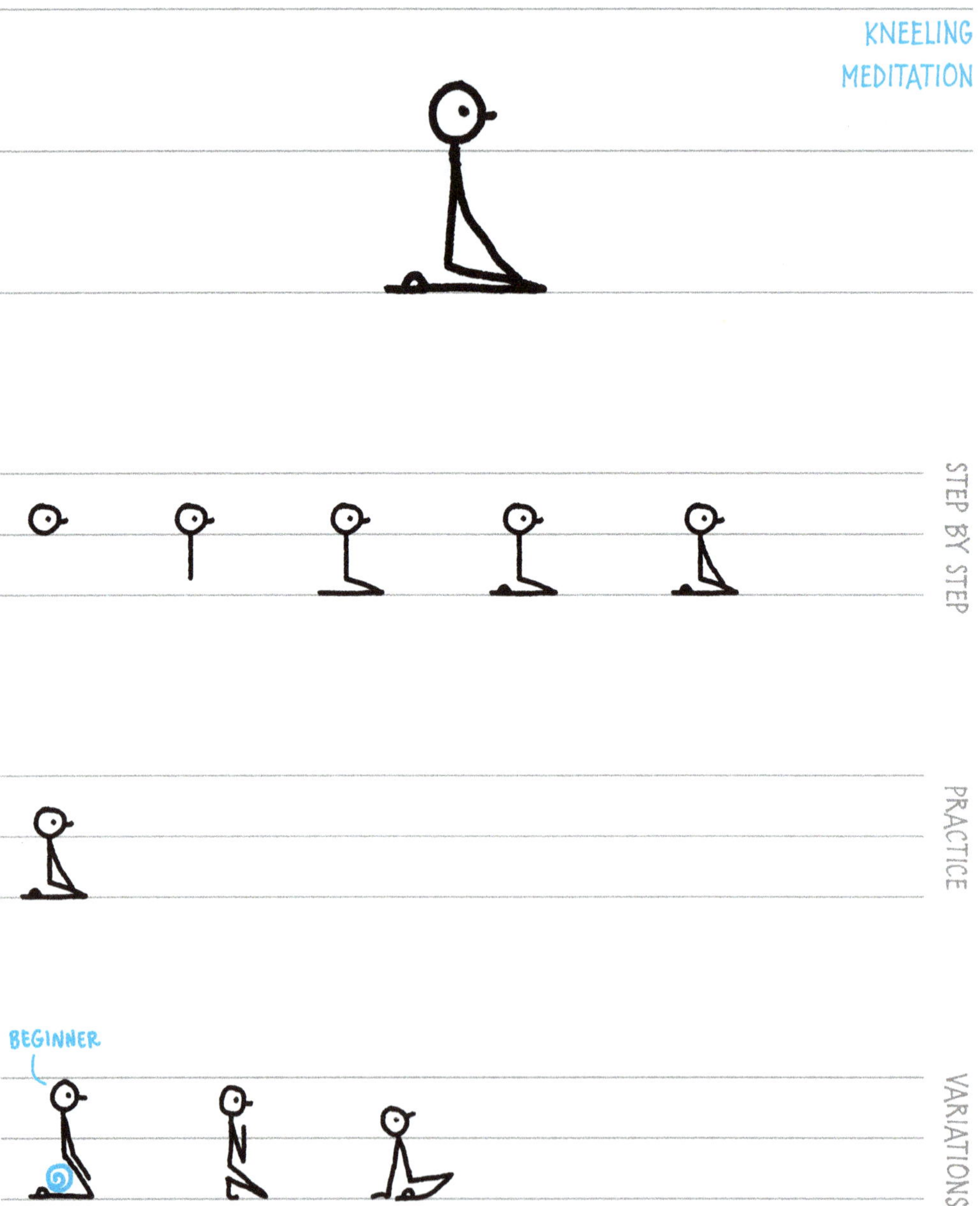

VIRASANA
HERO POSE

KNEELING
HIP OPENING

STEP BY STEP

PRACTICE

BEGINNER

SUPTA VIRASANA
(RECLINING HERO POSE)

VARIATIONS

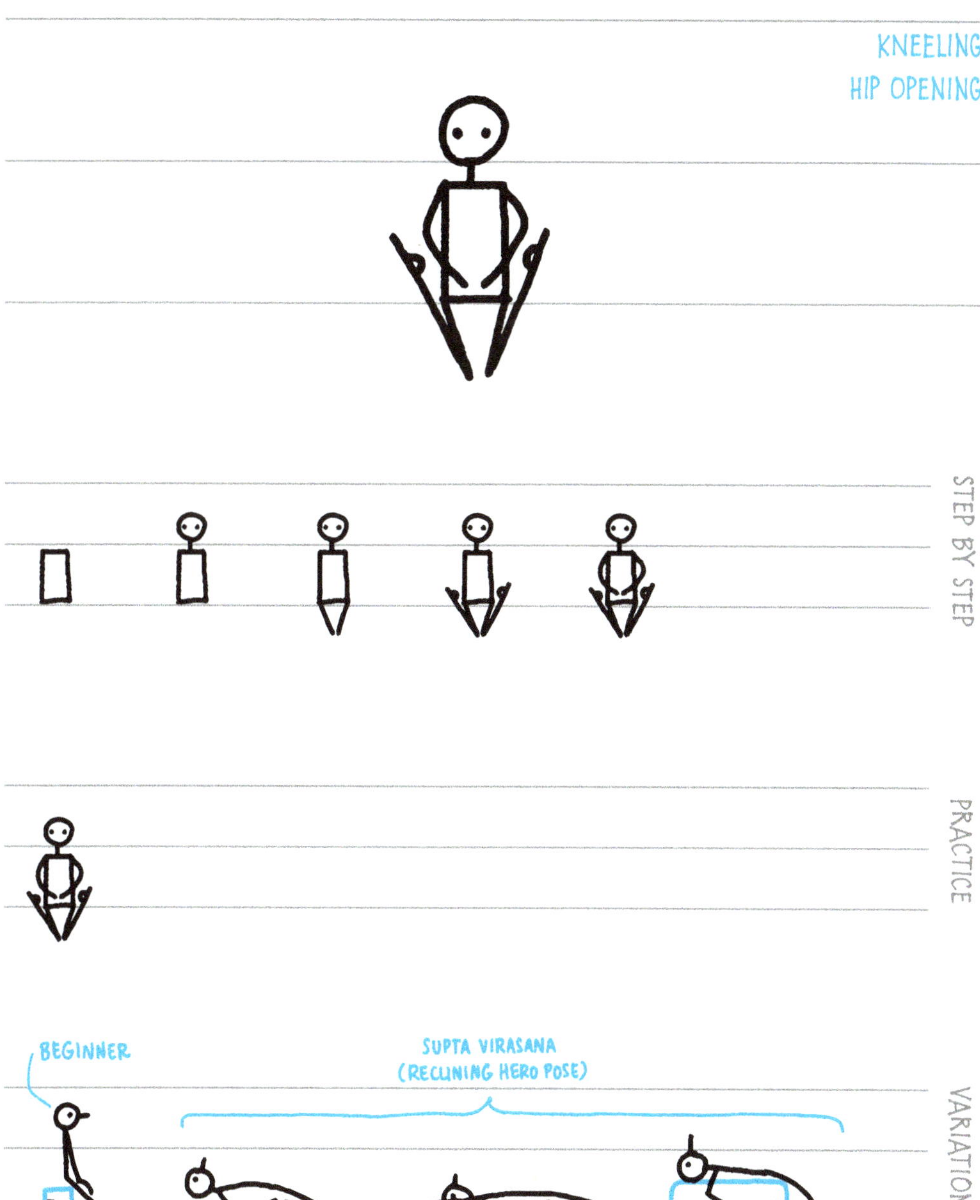

ADHO MUKHA VIRASANA

DOWNWARD FACING HERO POSE

KNEELING
SHOULDER OPENING

STEP BY STEP

PRACTICE

VARIATIONS

UTTHANA SHISHONASANA
(EXTENDED PUPPY POSE)

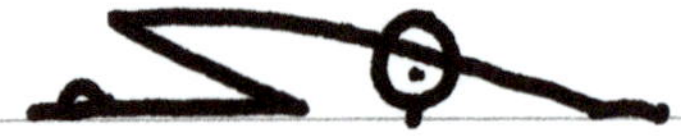

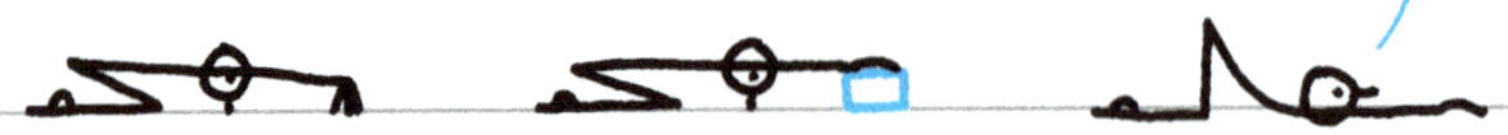

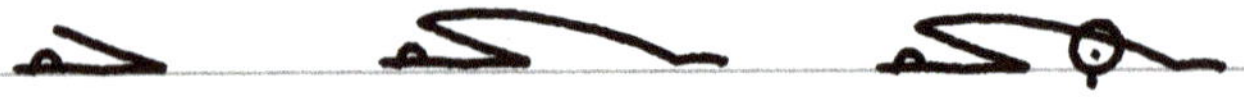

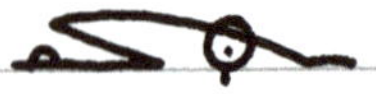

BALASANA

CHILD'S POSE

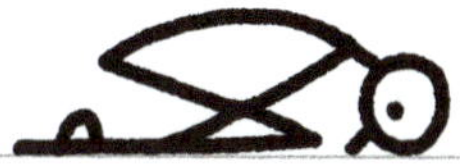

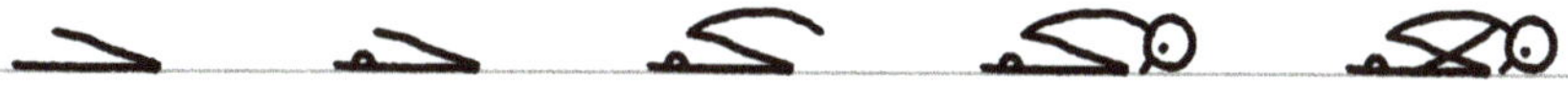

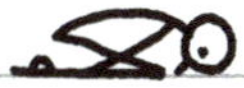

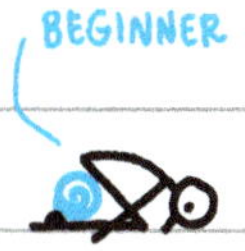

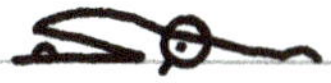

MARJARIASANA

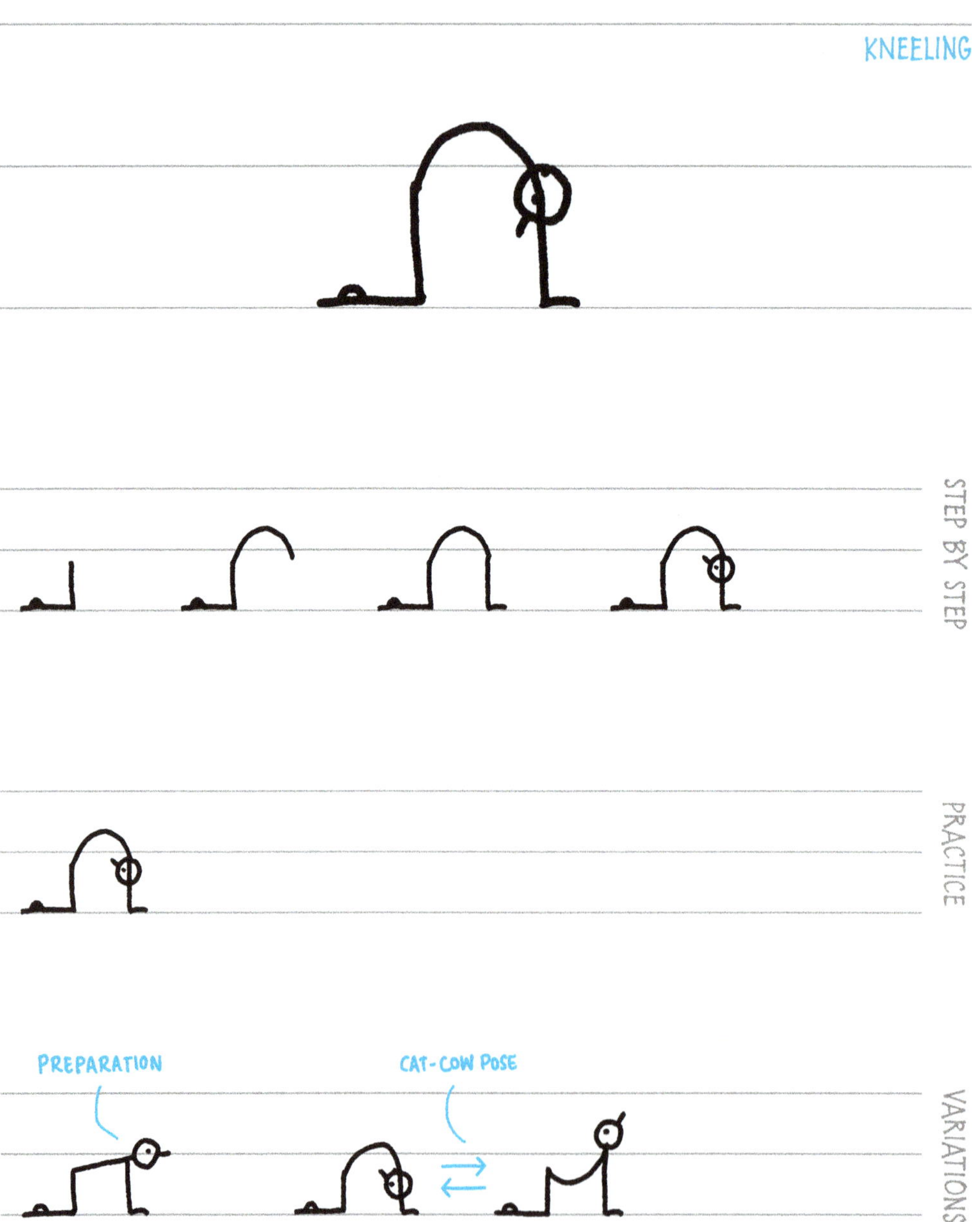

VYAGHRASANA
TIGER POSE

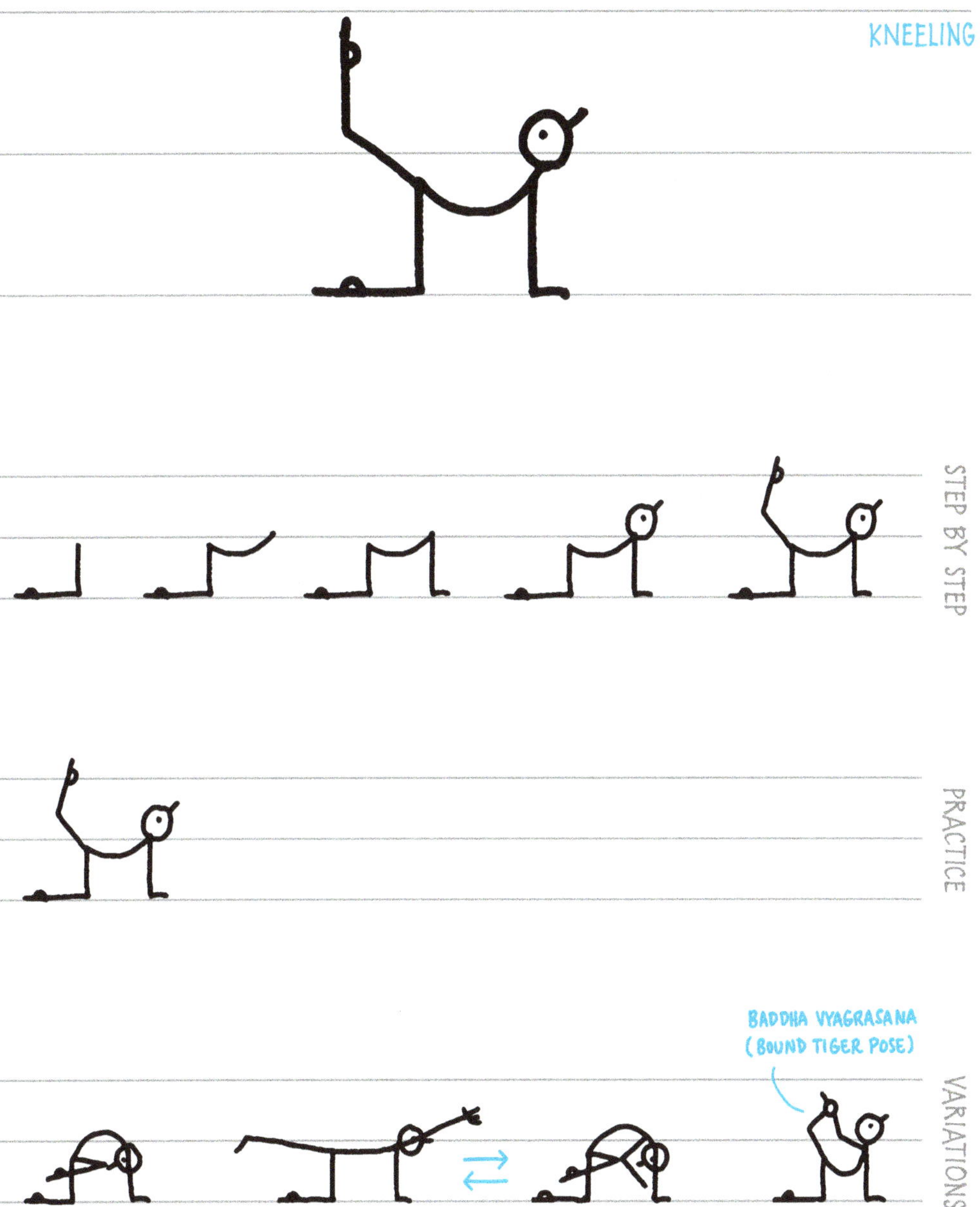

USTRASANA
CAMEL POSE

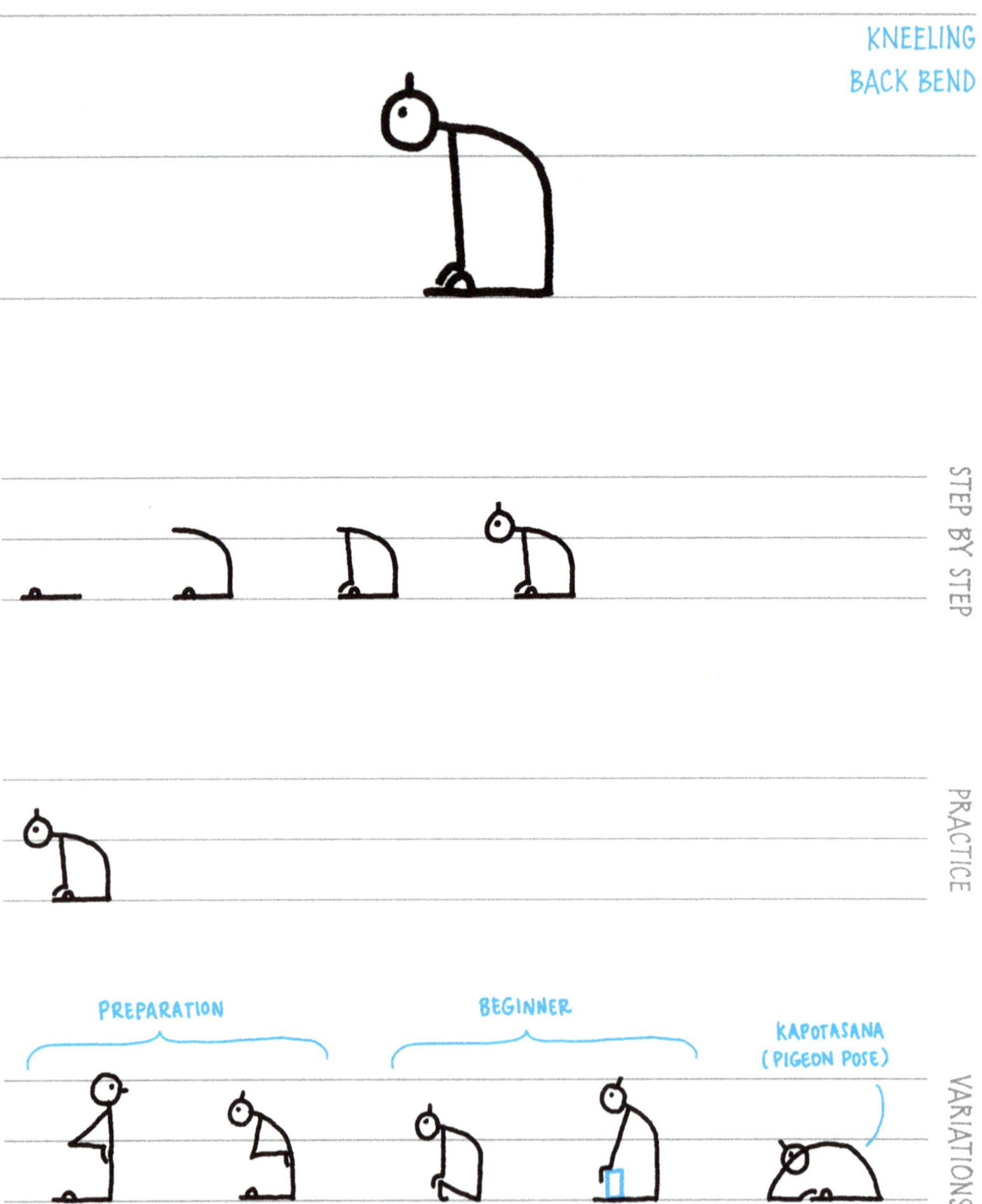

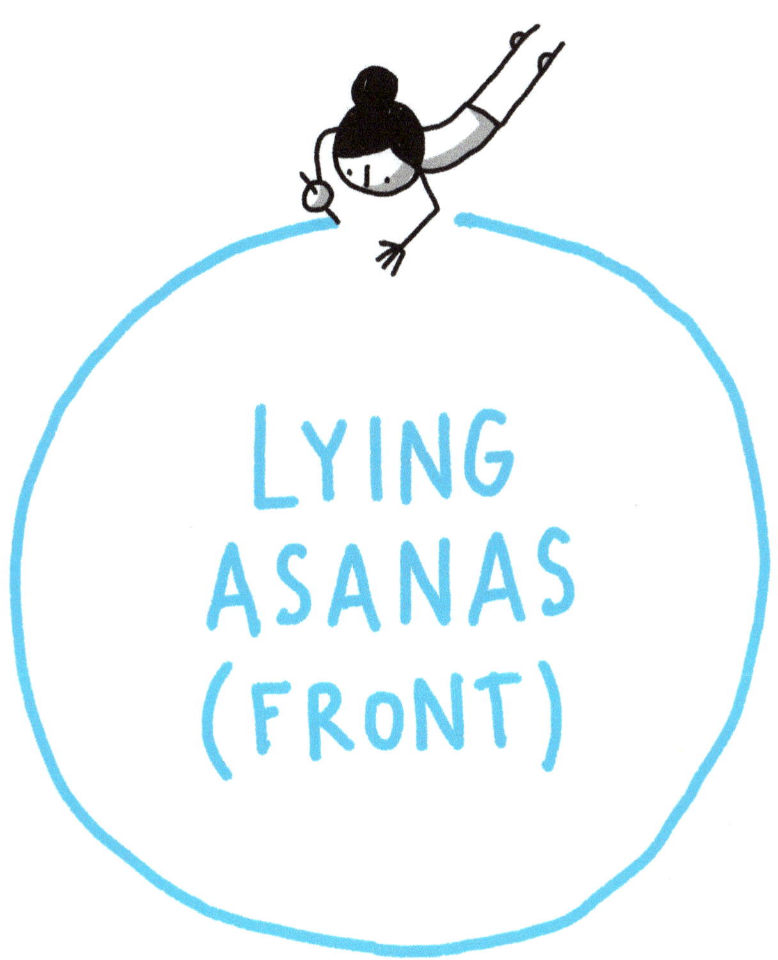

LYING
ASANAS
(FRONT)

BHUJANGASANA

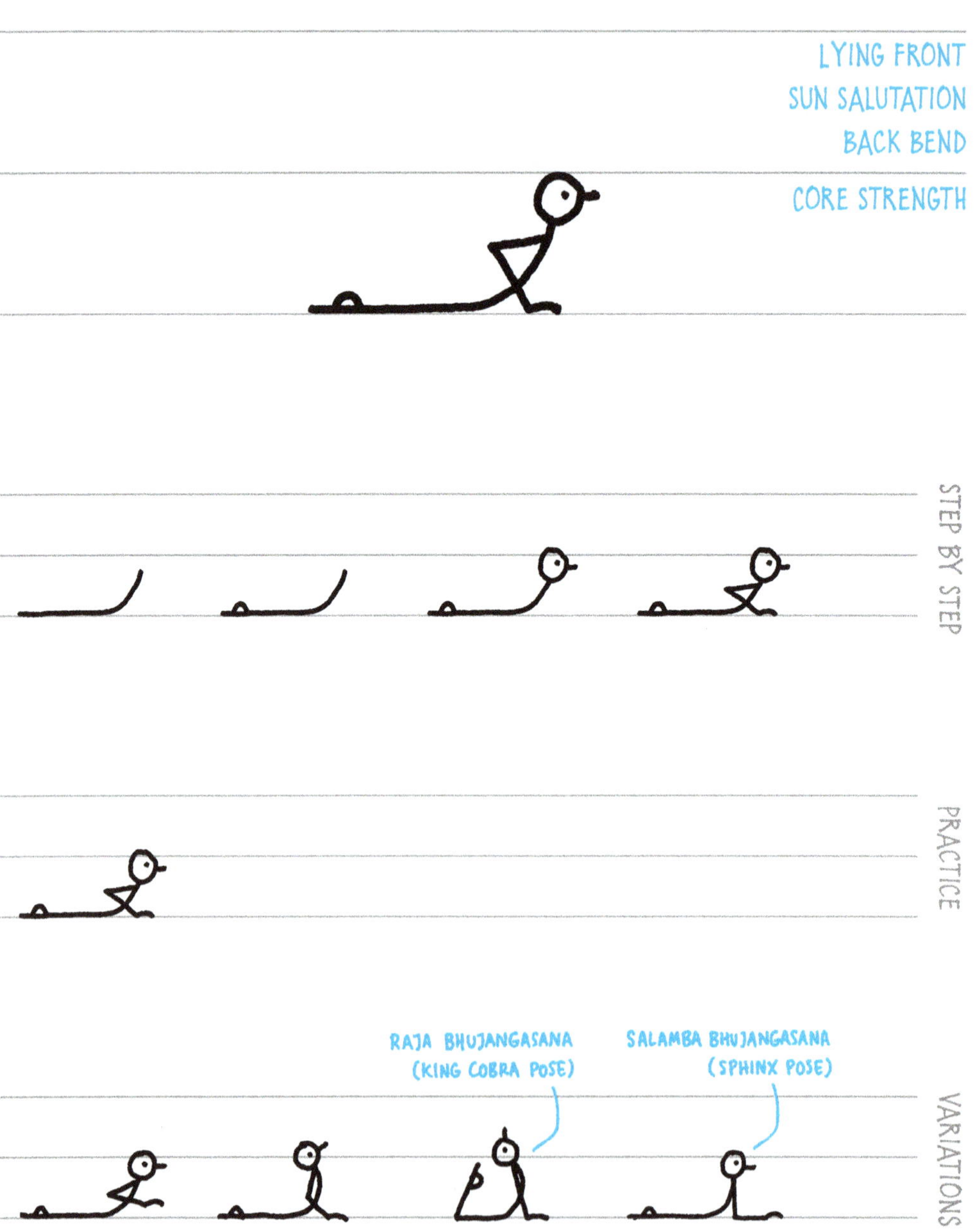

SALABHASANA

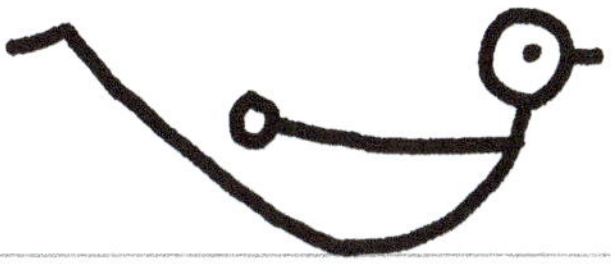

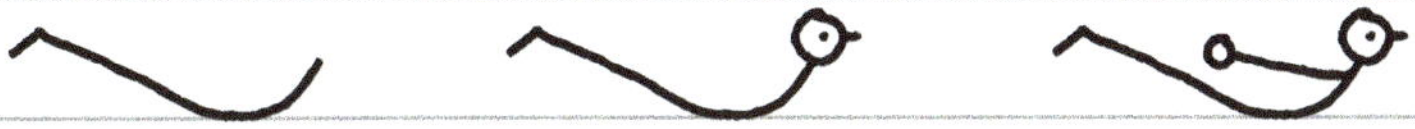

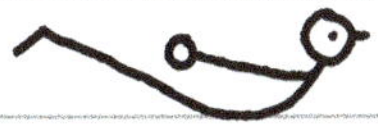

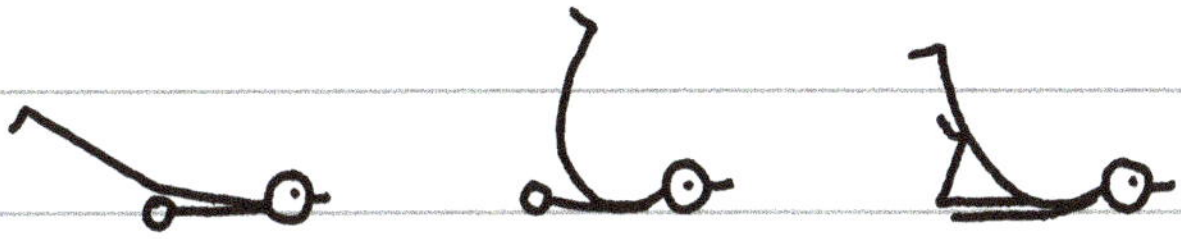

VIPARITA SHALABHASANA

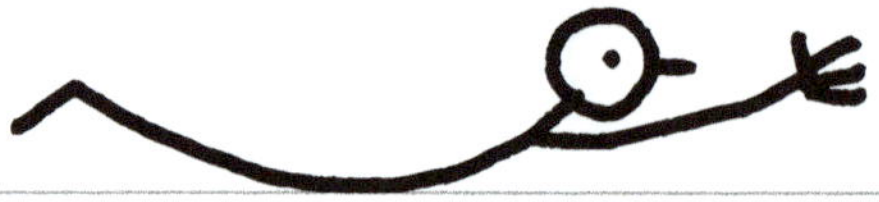

STEP BY STEP

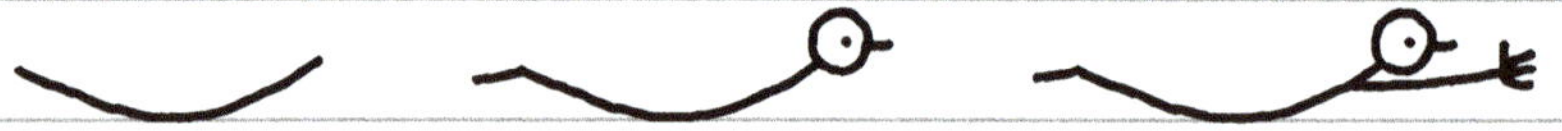

PRACTICE

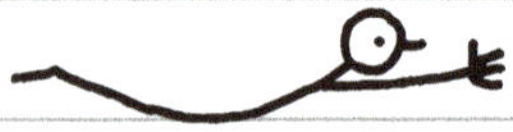

VARIATIONS

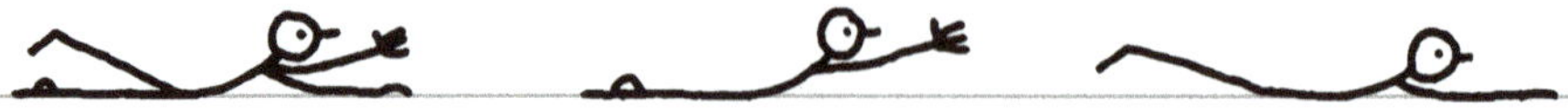

DHANURASANA

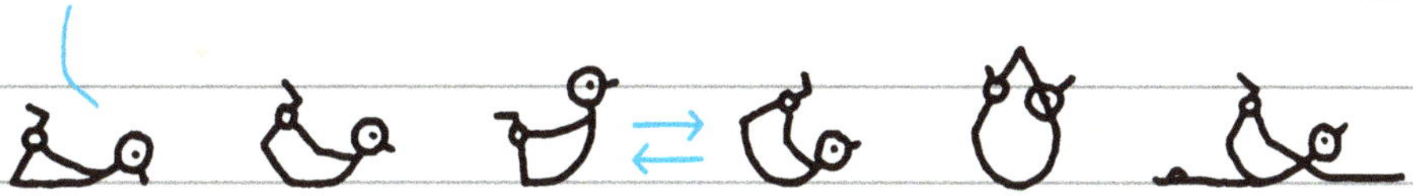

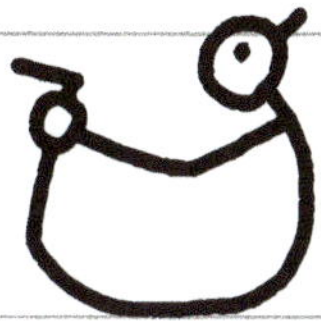

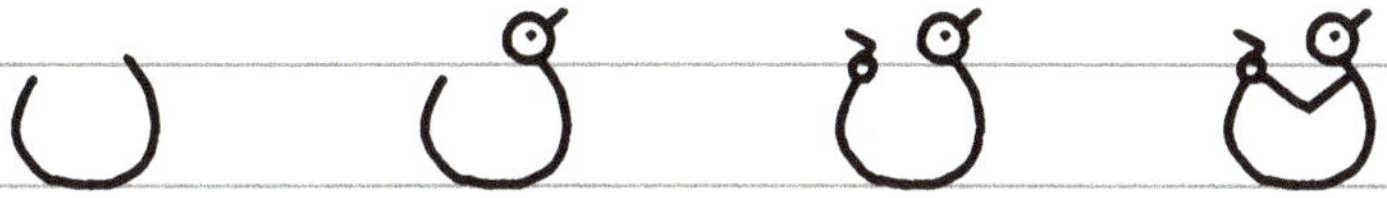

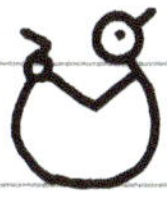

MAKRASANA

CROCODILE POSE

LYING FRONT
RESTORATIVE

STEP BY STEP

PRACTICE

VARIATIONS

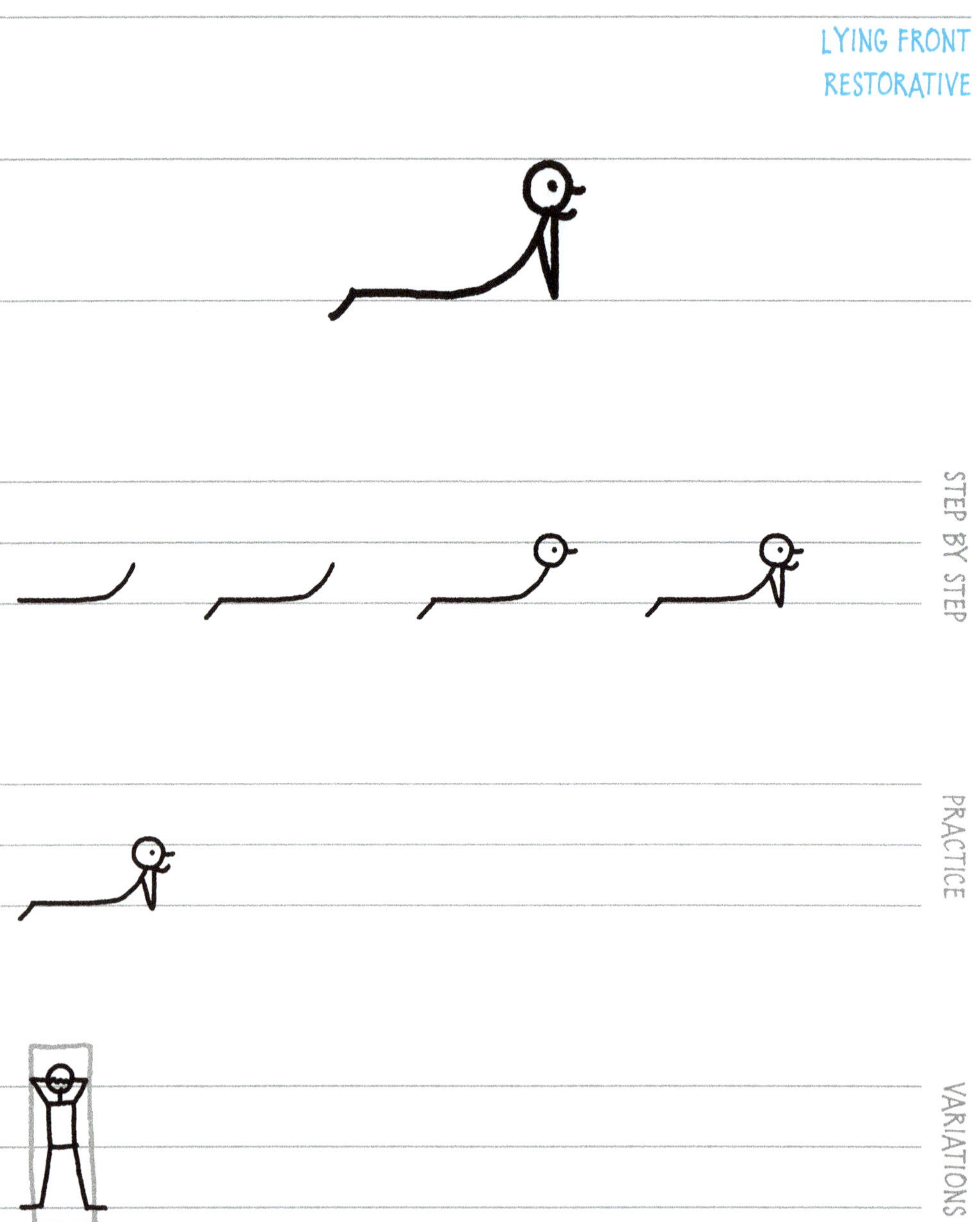

BHEKASANA

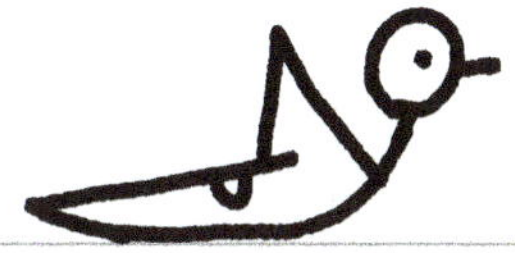

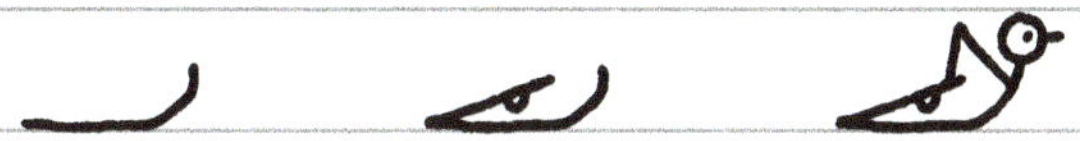

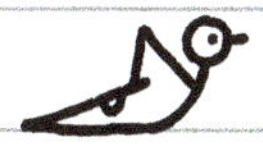

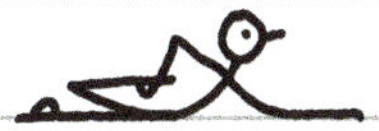

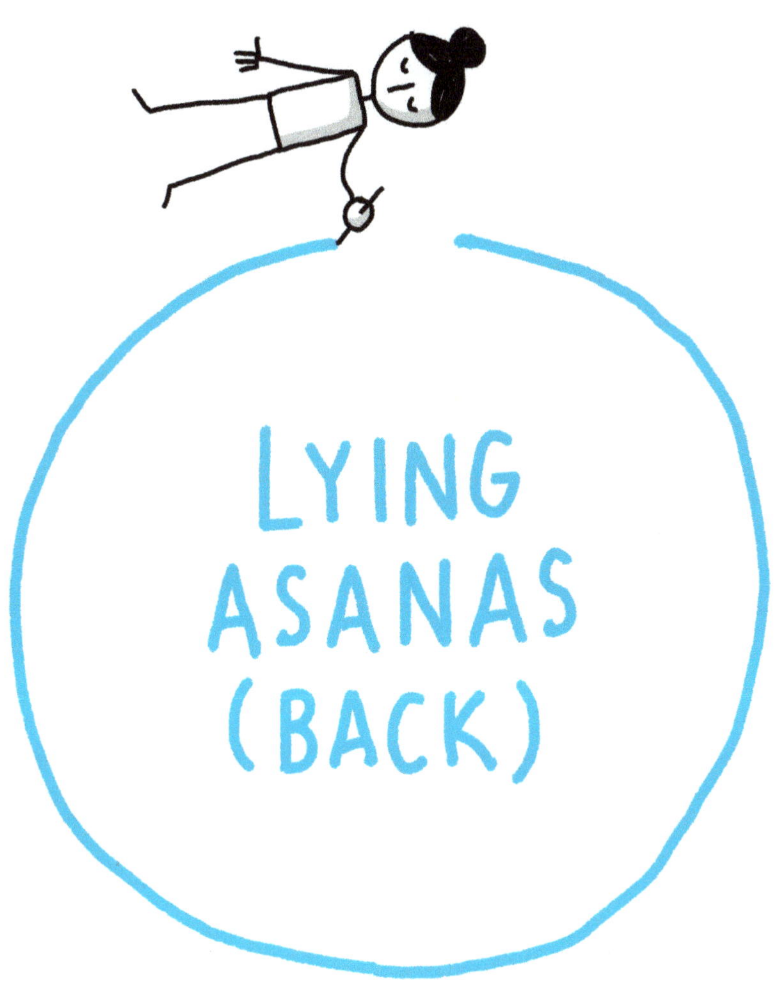
LYING
ASANAS
(BACK)

SAVASANA
CORPSE POSE

LYING BACK
RESTORATIVE

STEP BY STEP

PRACTICE

SUPTA BADDHAKONASANA
(RECLINING BUTTERFLY)

VARIATIONS

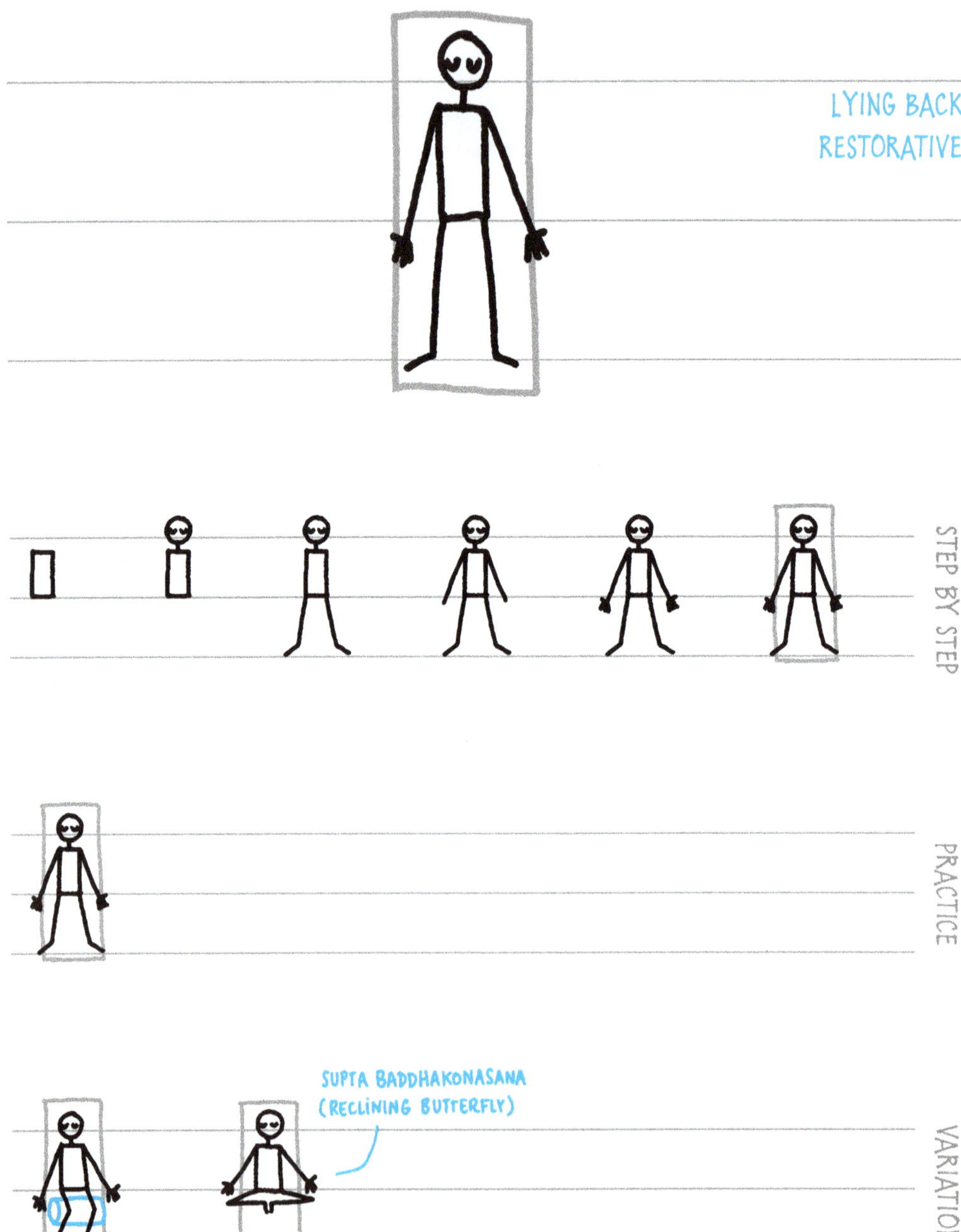

PREPARATION FOR SAVASANA
WHOLE BODY TENSING

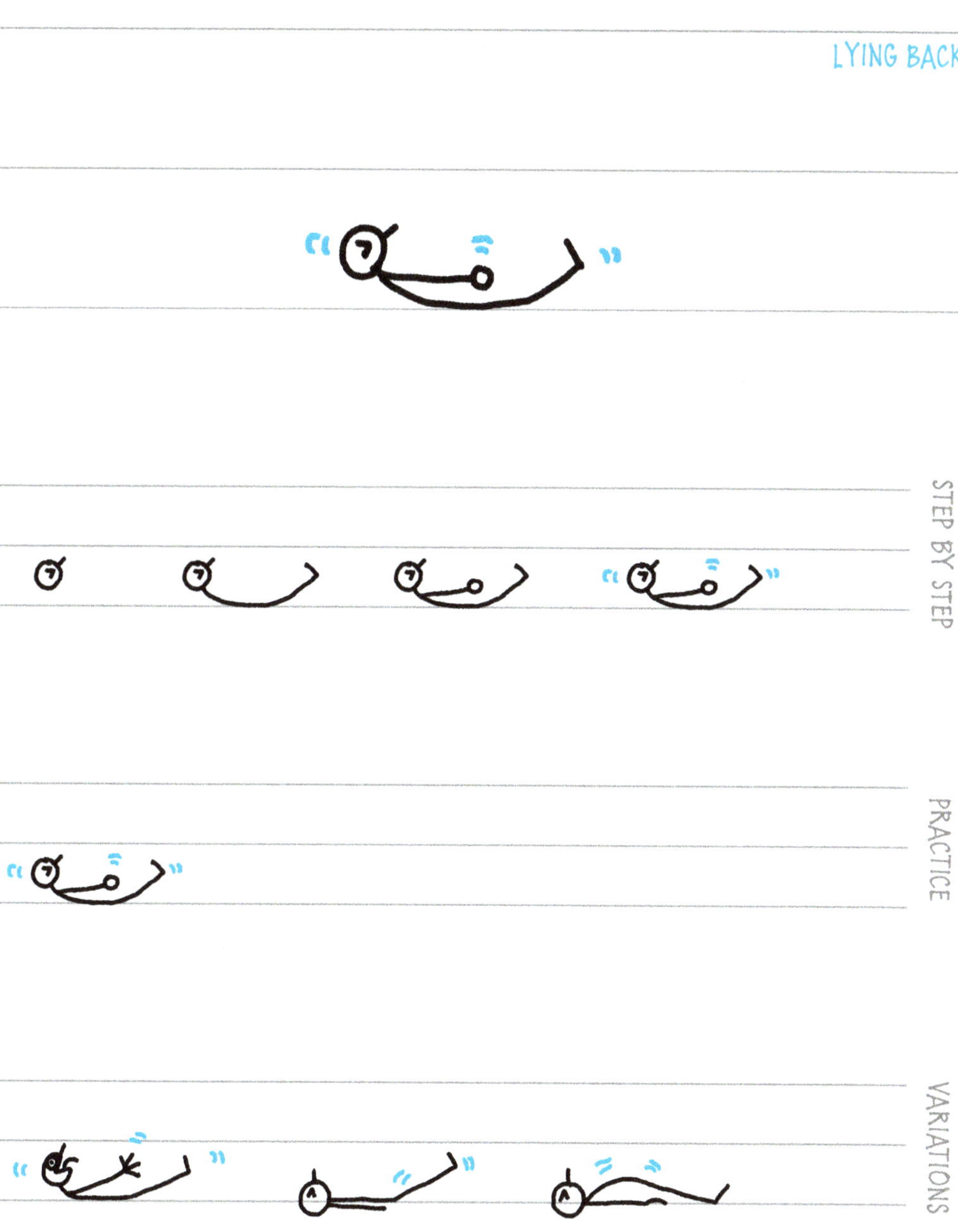

APANASANA

KNEES-TO-CHEST POSE

LYING BACK
RESTORATIVE

STEP BY STEP

PRACTICE

VARIATIONS

ANANDA BALASANA
(HAPPY BABY POSE)

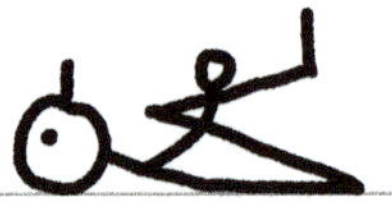

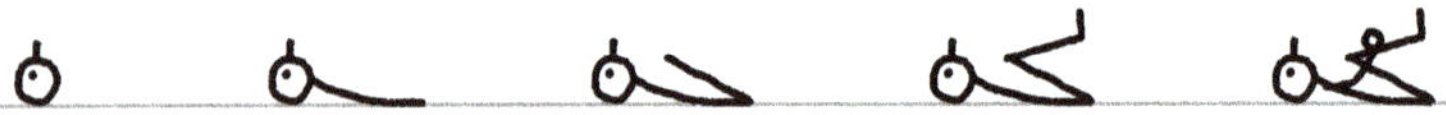

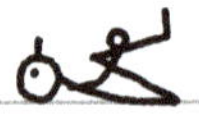

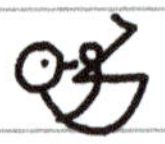

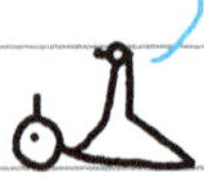

SUPTA KAPOTASANA

RECLINING PIGEON POSE

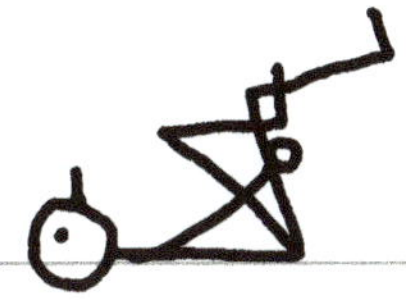

STEP BY STEP

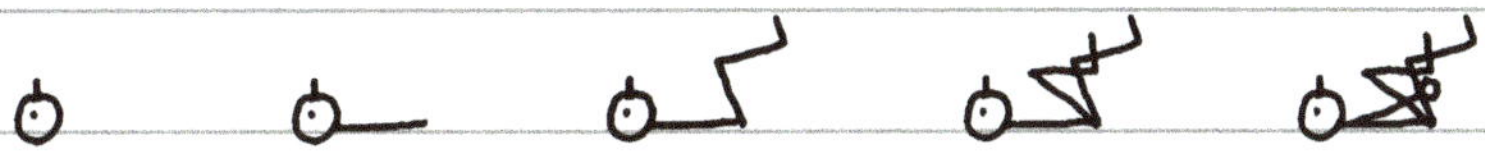

PRACTICE

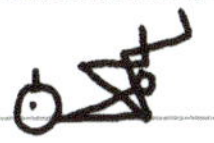

VARIATIONS

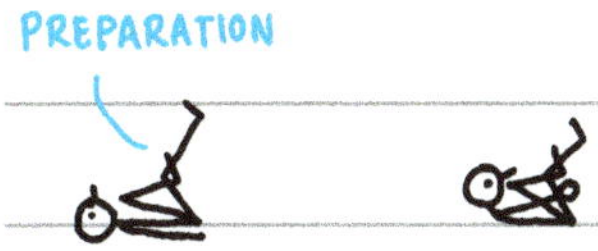

PREPARATION

SUPTA PADANGUSTHASANA

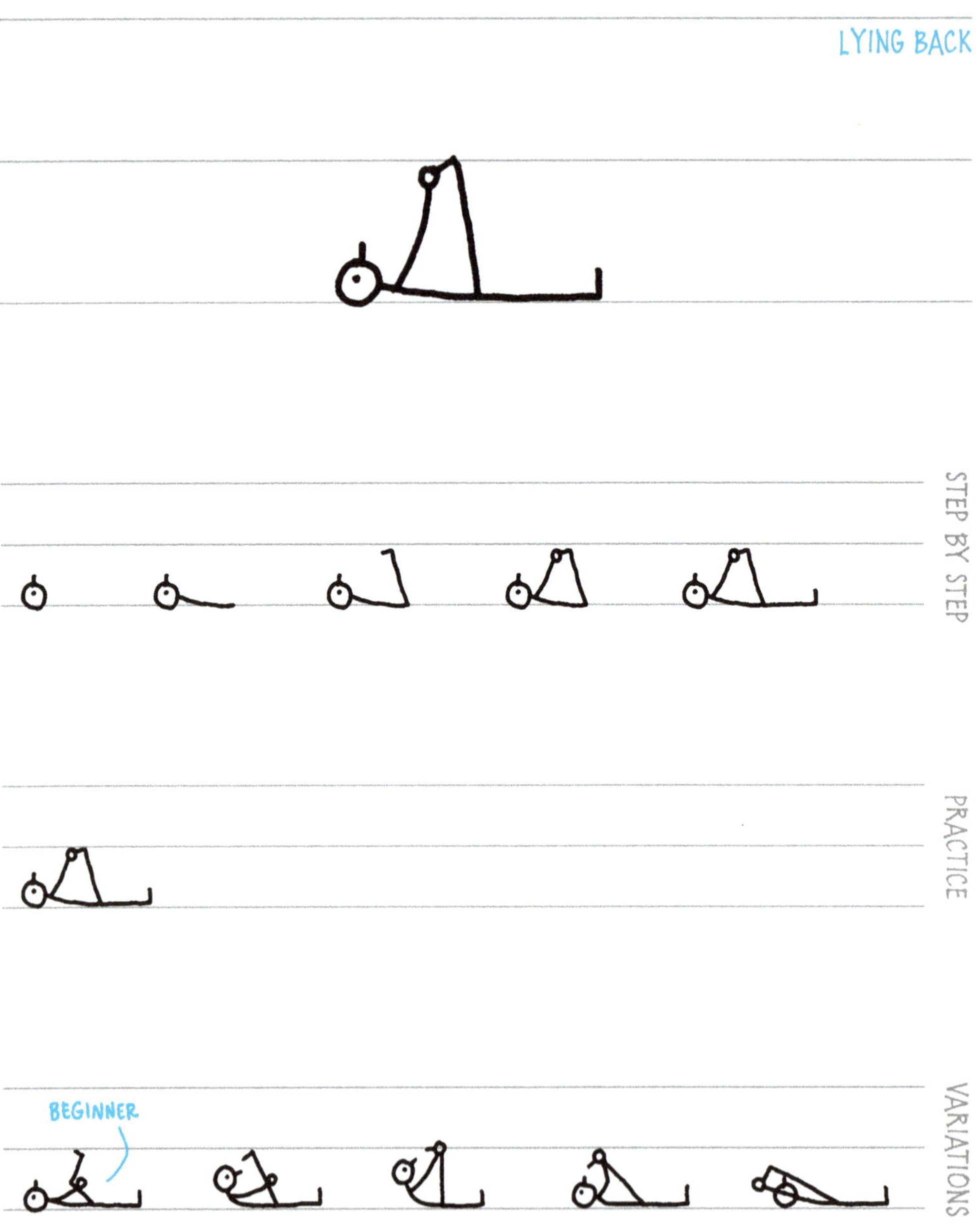

SUPTA MATSYENDRASANA

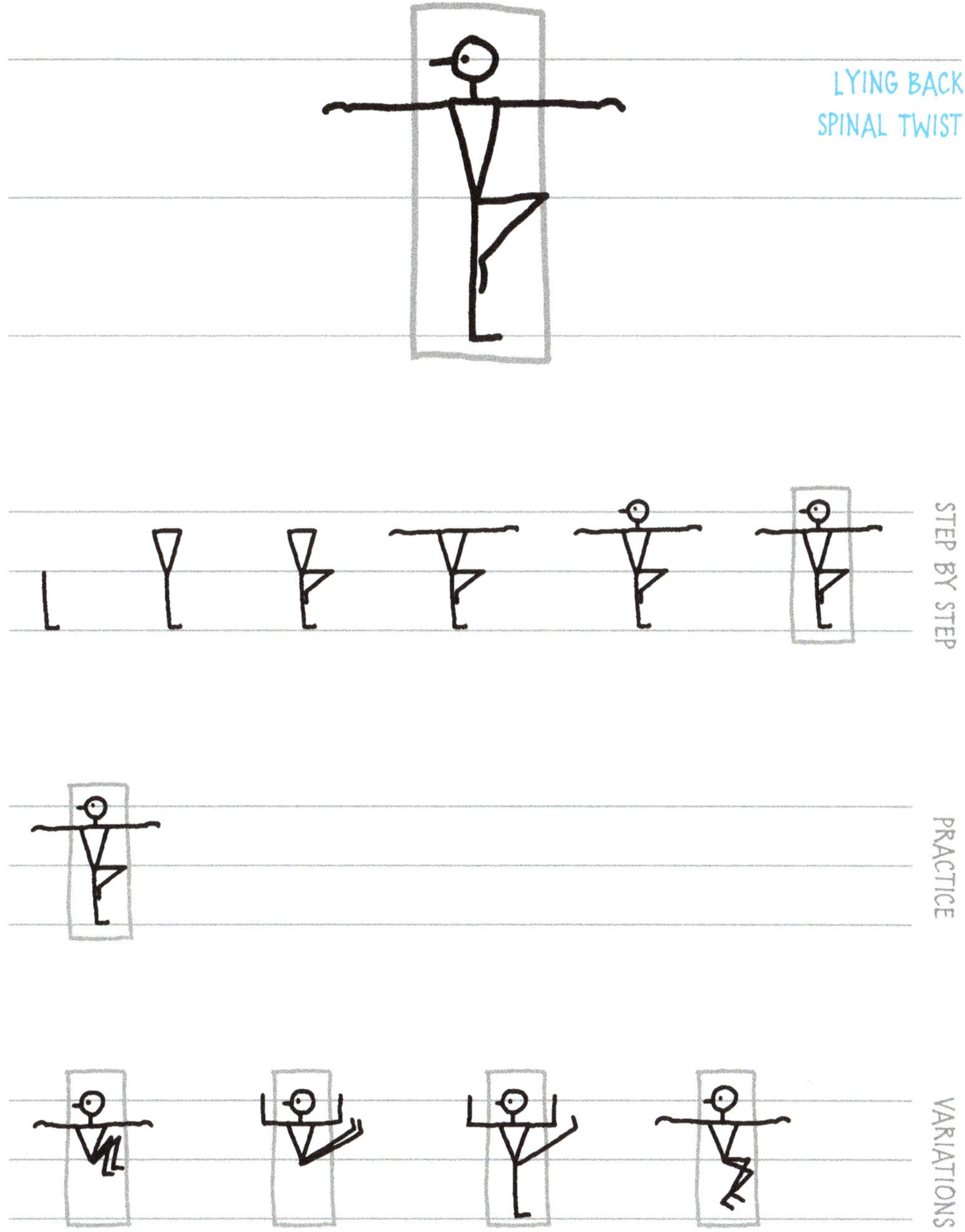

UTTANPADASANA

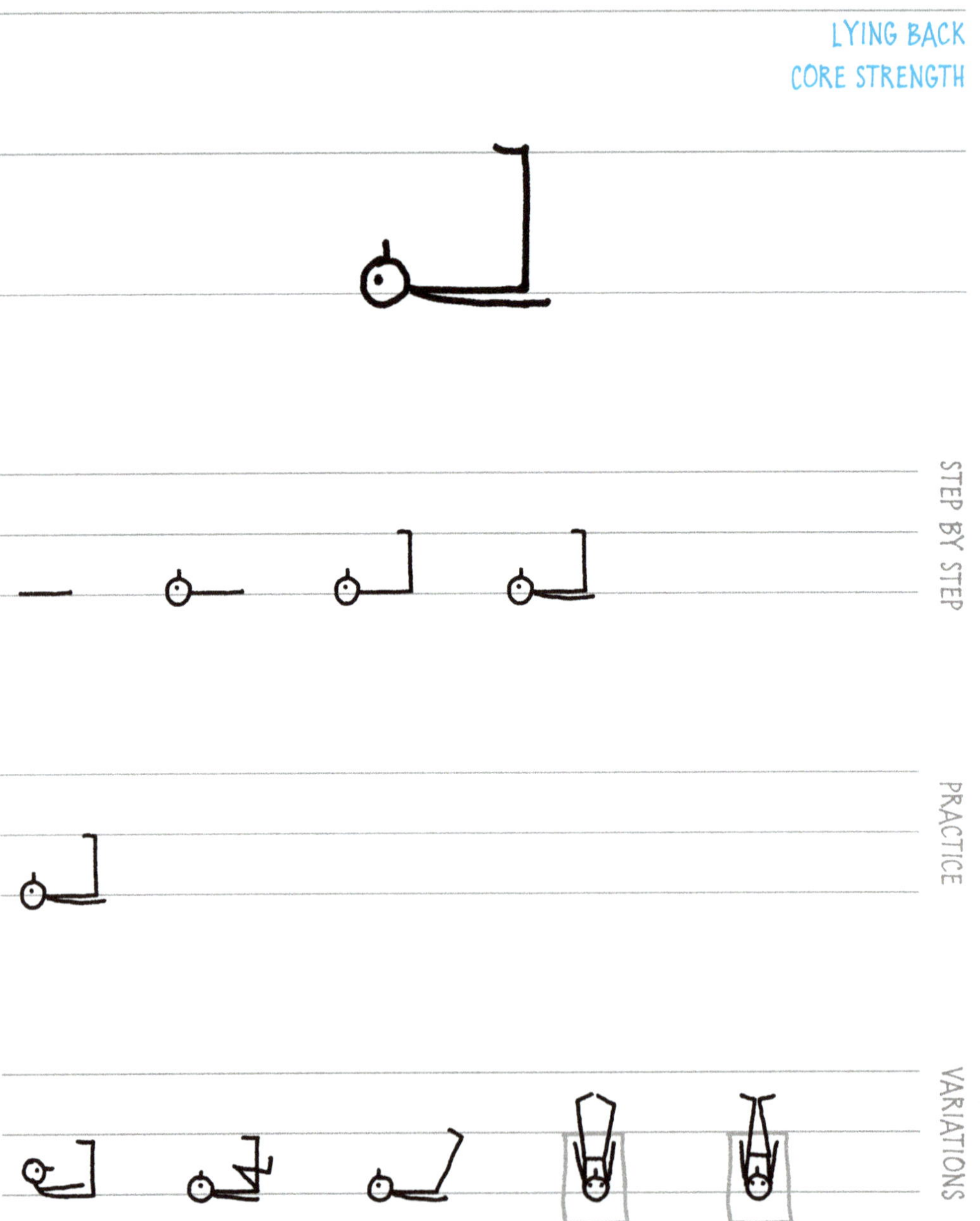

EKA PADA UTTANPADASANA
SINGLE LEG RAISED POSE

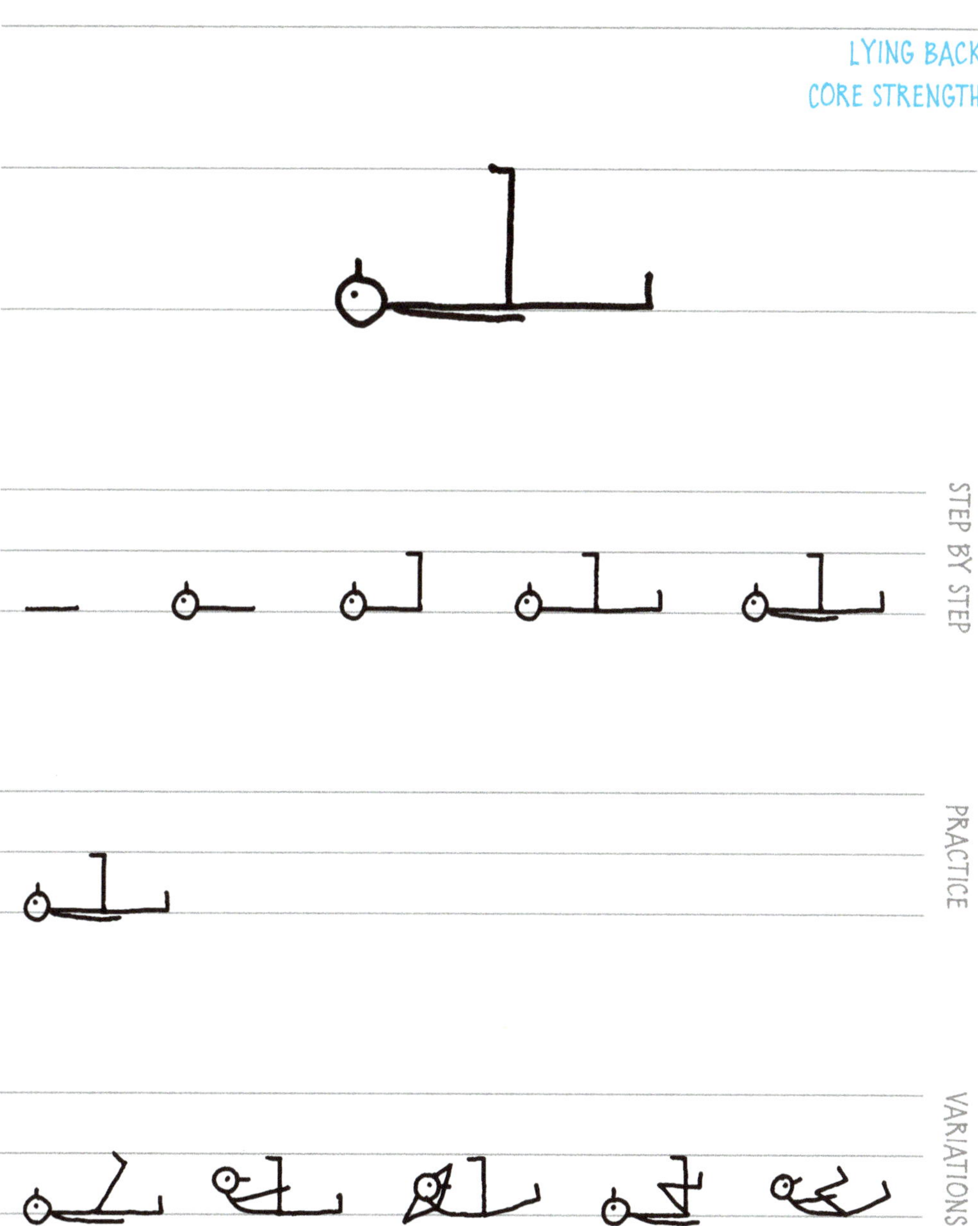

HALASANA

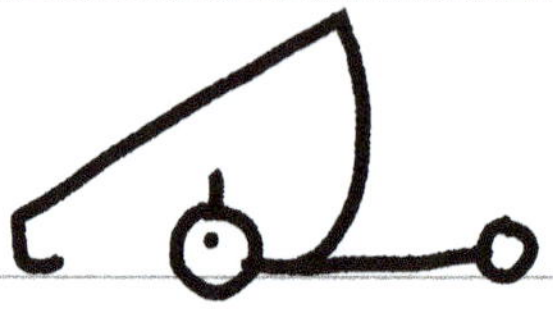

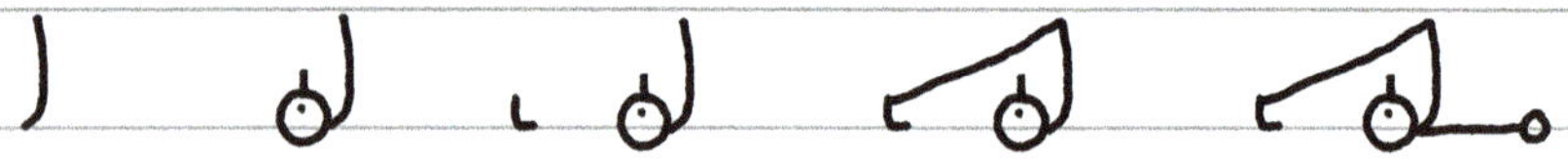

STEP BY STEP

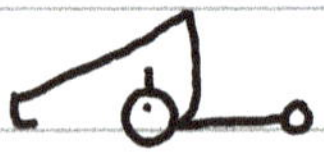

PRACTICE

BEGINNER

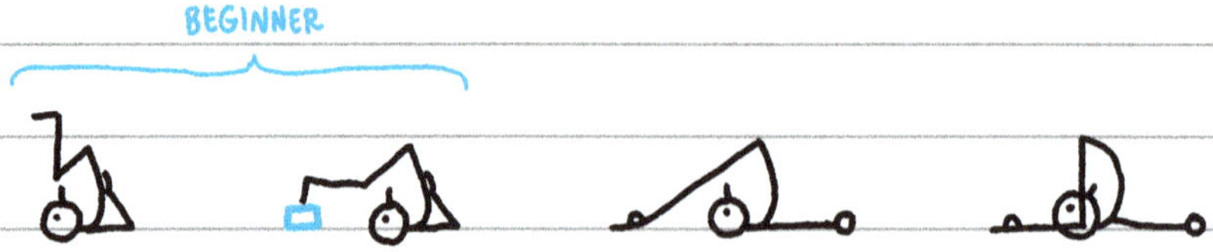

VARIATIONS

MATSYASANA

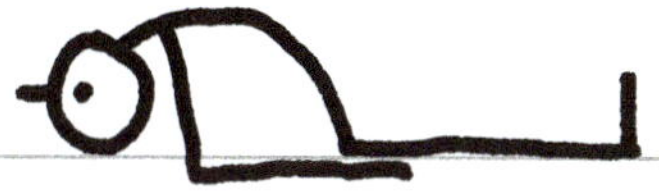

STEP BY STEP

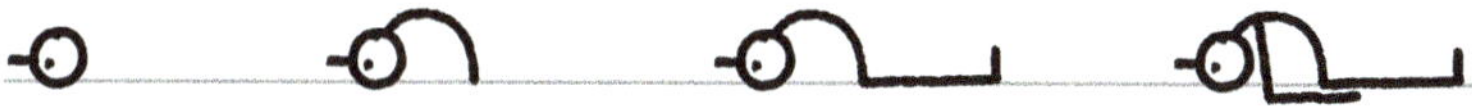

PRACTICE

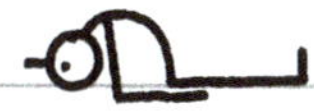

VARIATIONS

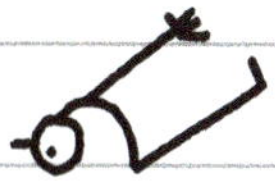

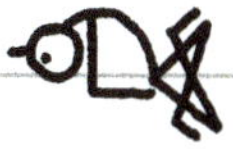

SETU BANDHA SARVANGASANA

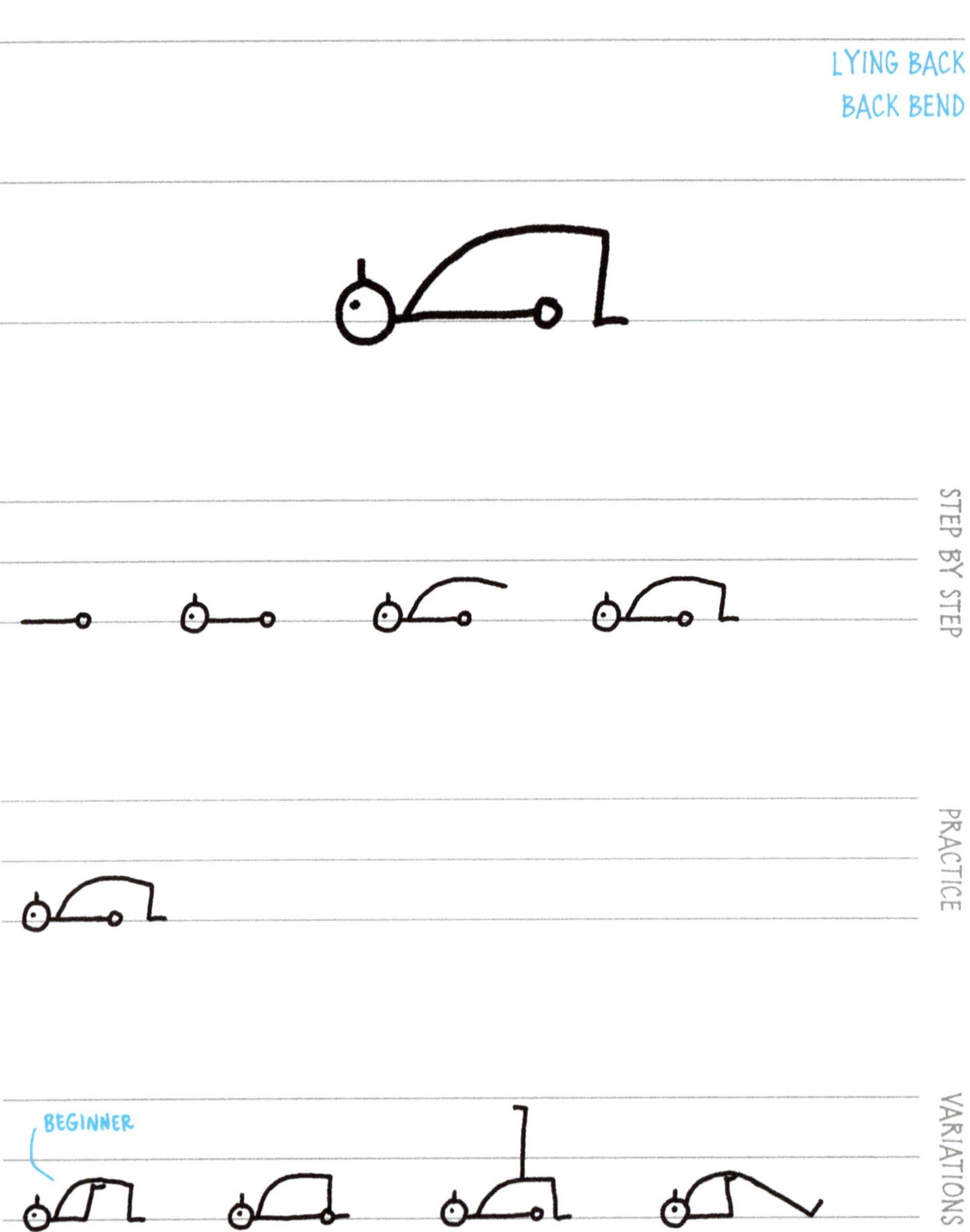

CHAKRASANA

WHEEL POSE

LYING BACK
BACK BEND
STEP BY STEP
PRACTICE
PREPARATION
VARIATIONS

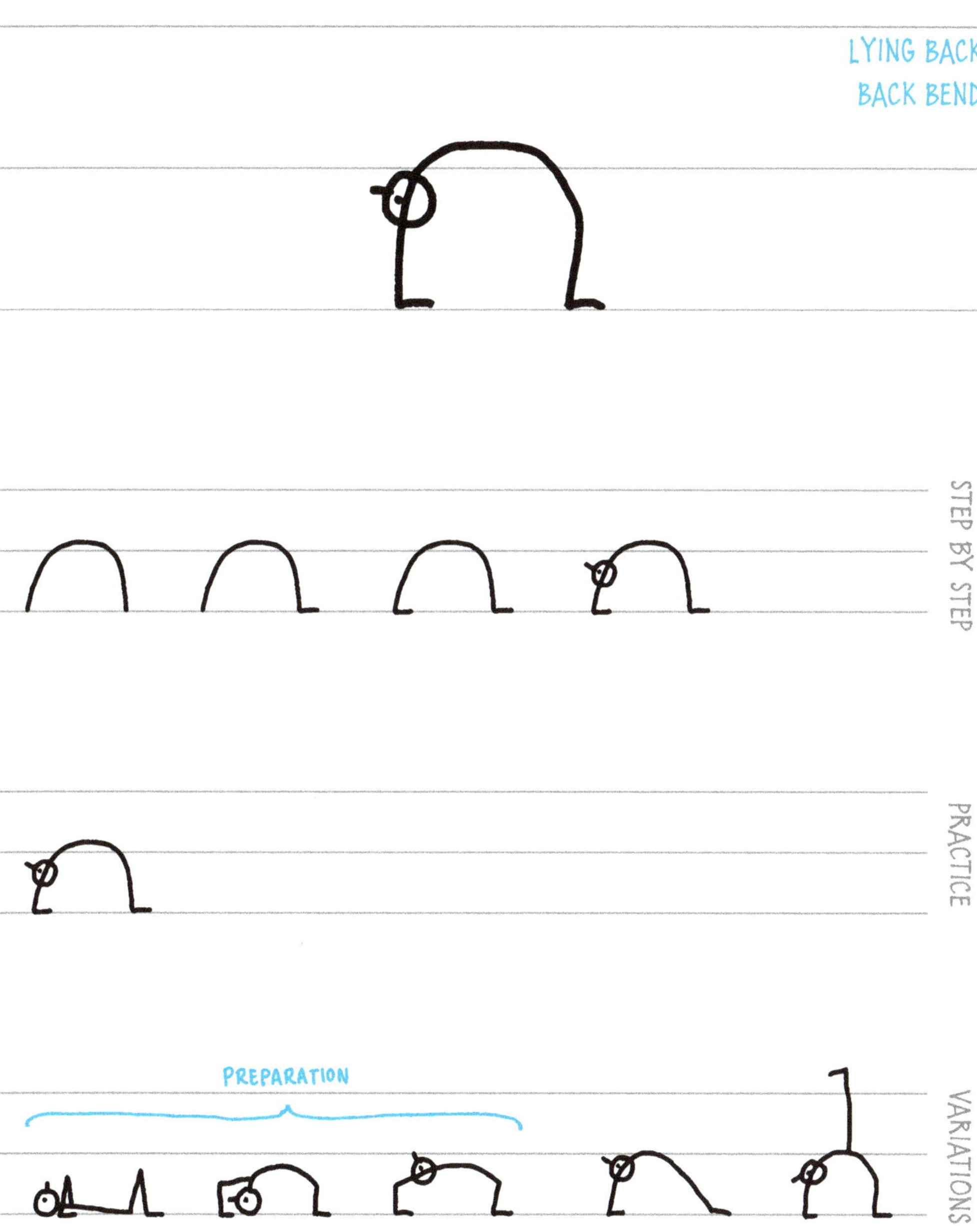

YOGA NIDRASANA

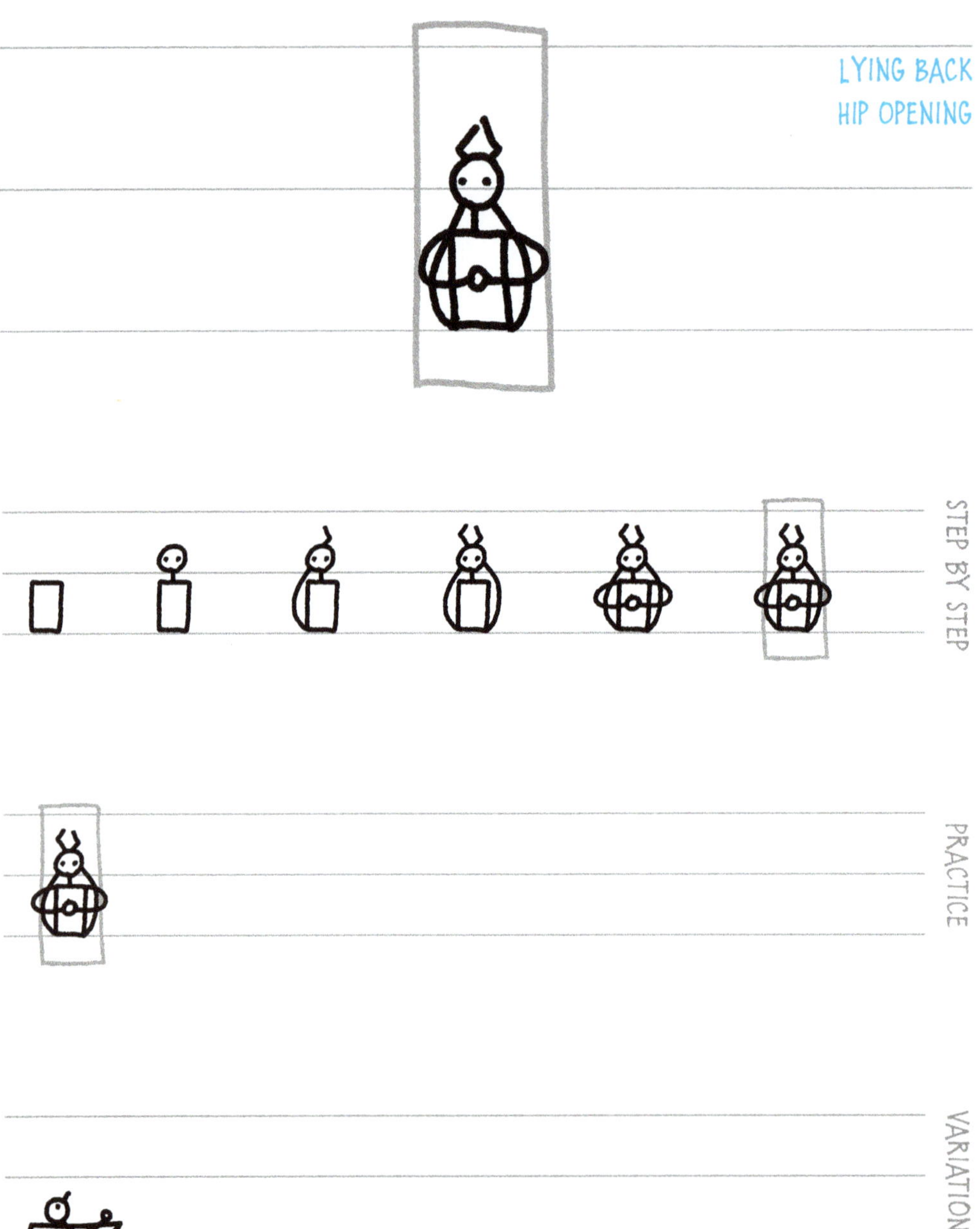

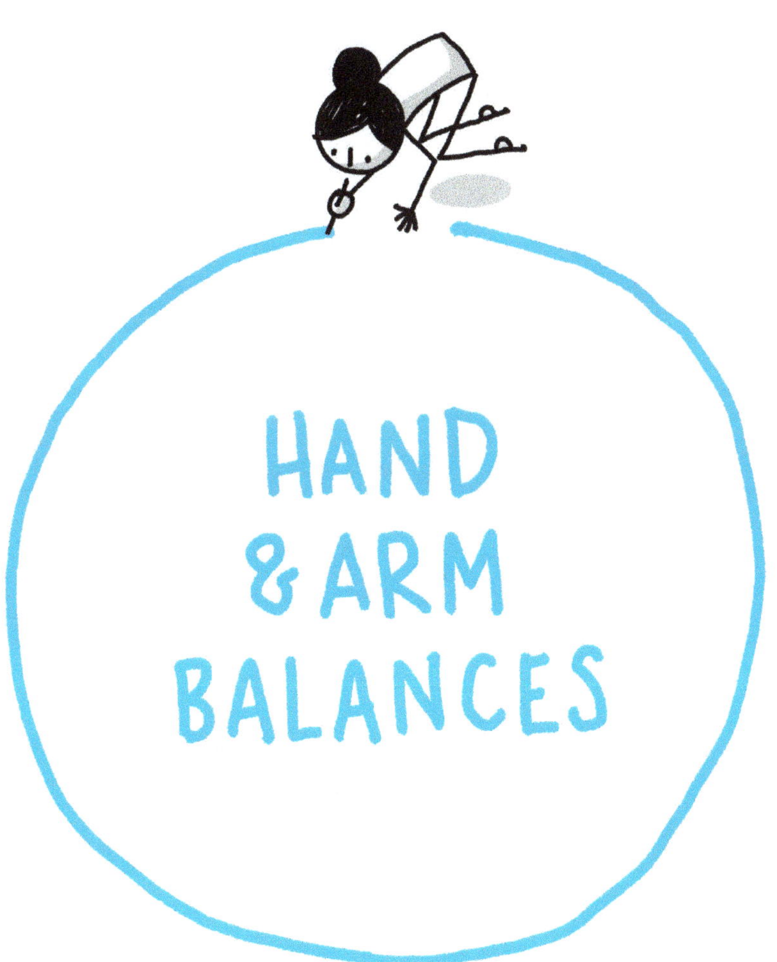

HAND
& ARM
BALANCES

KUMBHAKASANA
PLANK

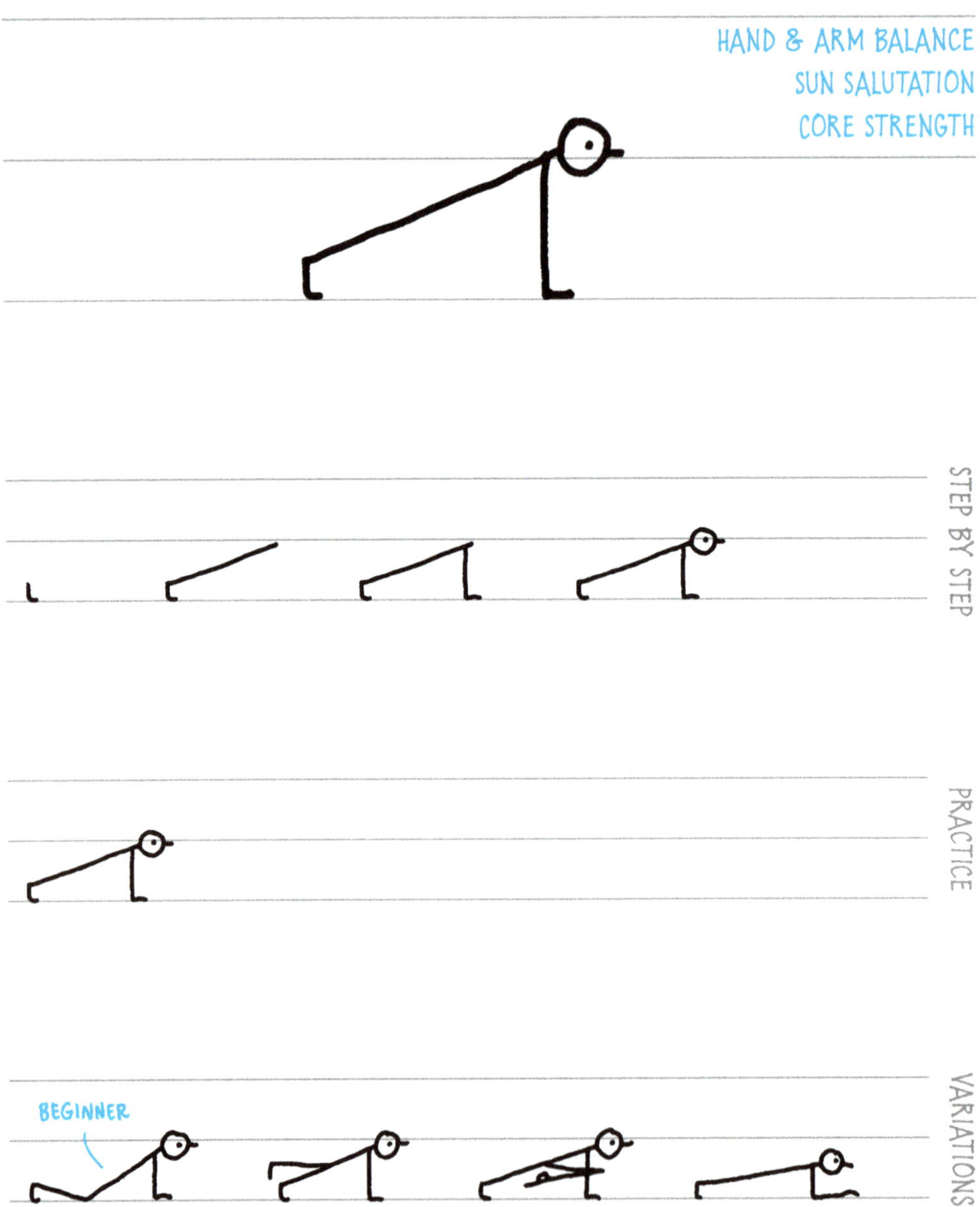

VASISTHASANA

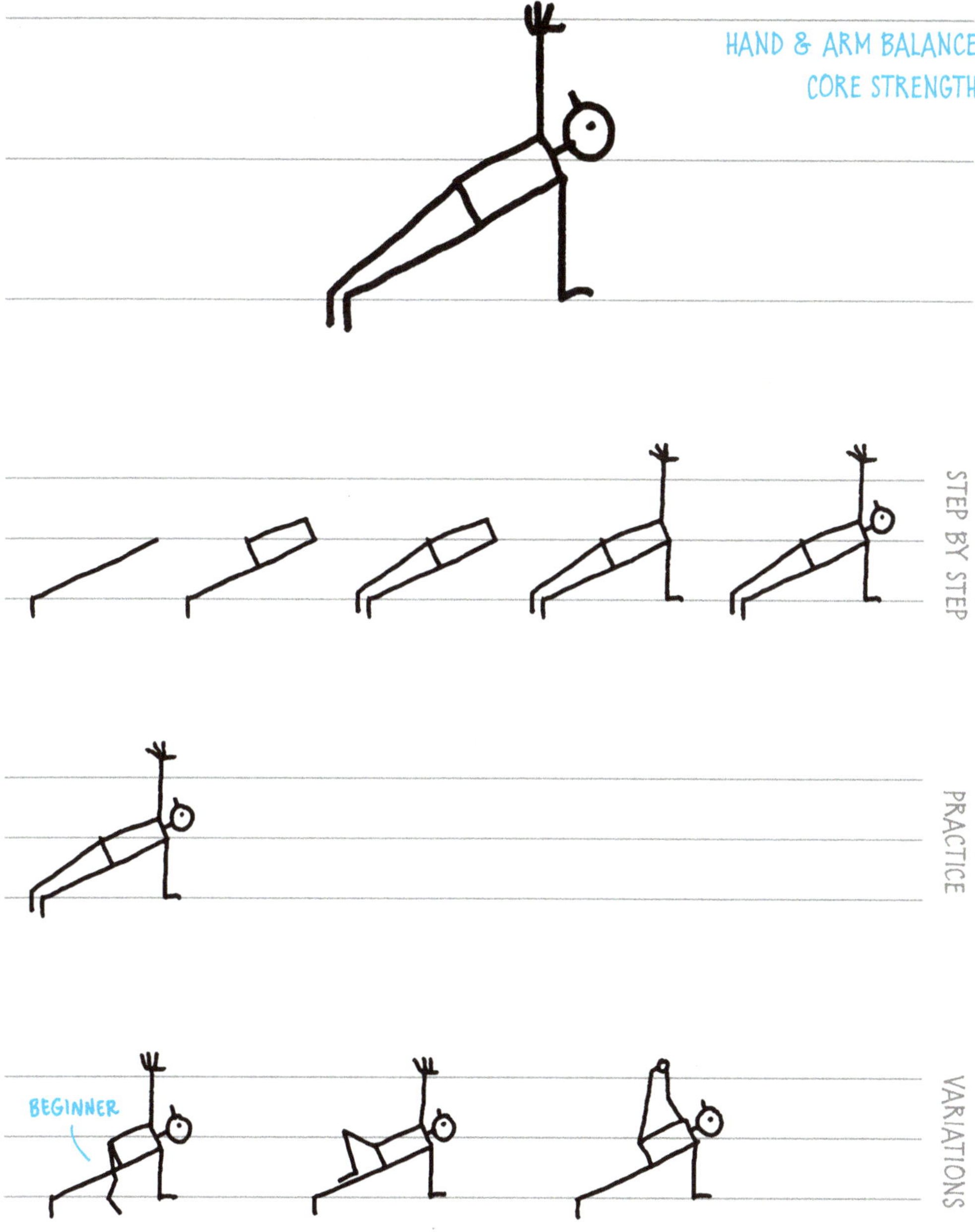

CHATURANGA DANDASANA
FOUR-LIMBED STAFF POSE

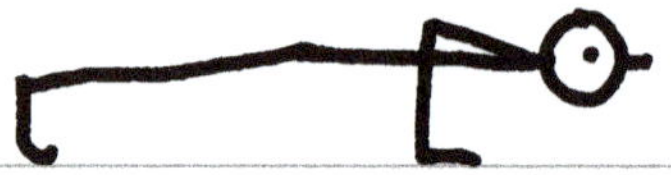

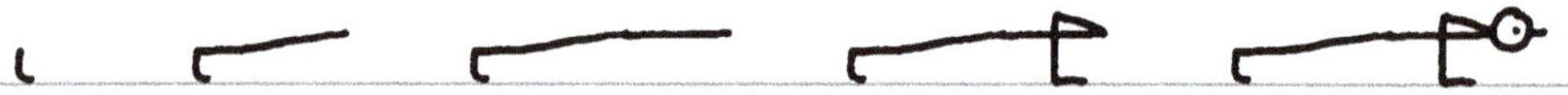

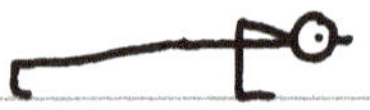

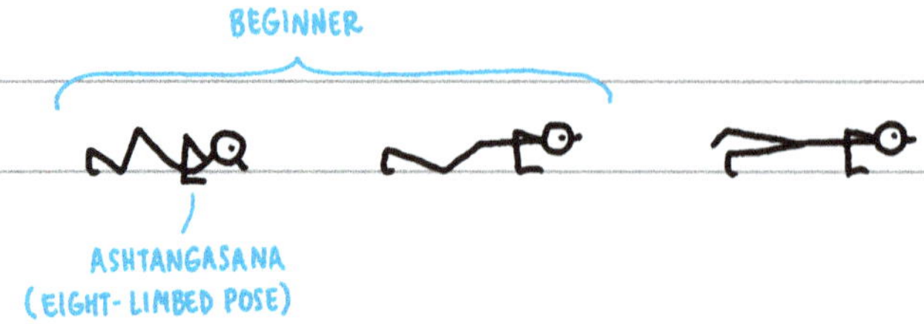

URDHVA MUKHA SVANASANA
UPWARD FACING DOG

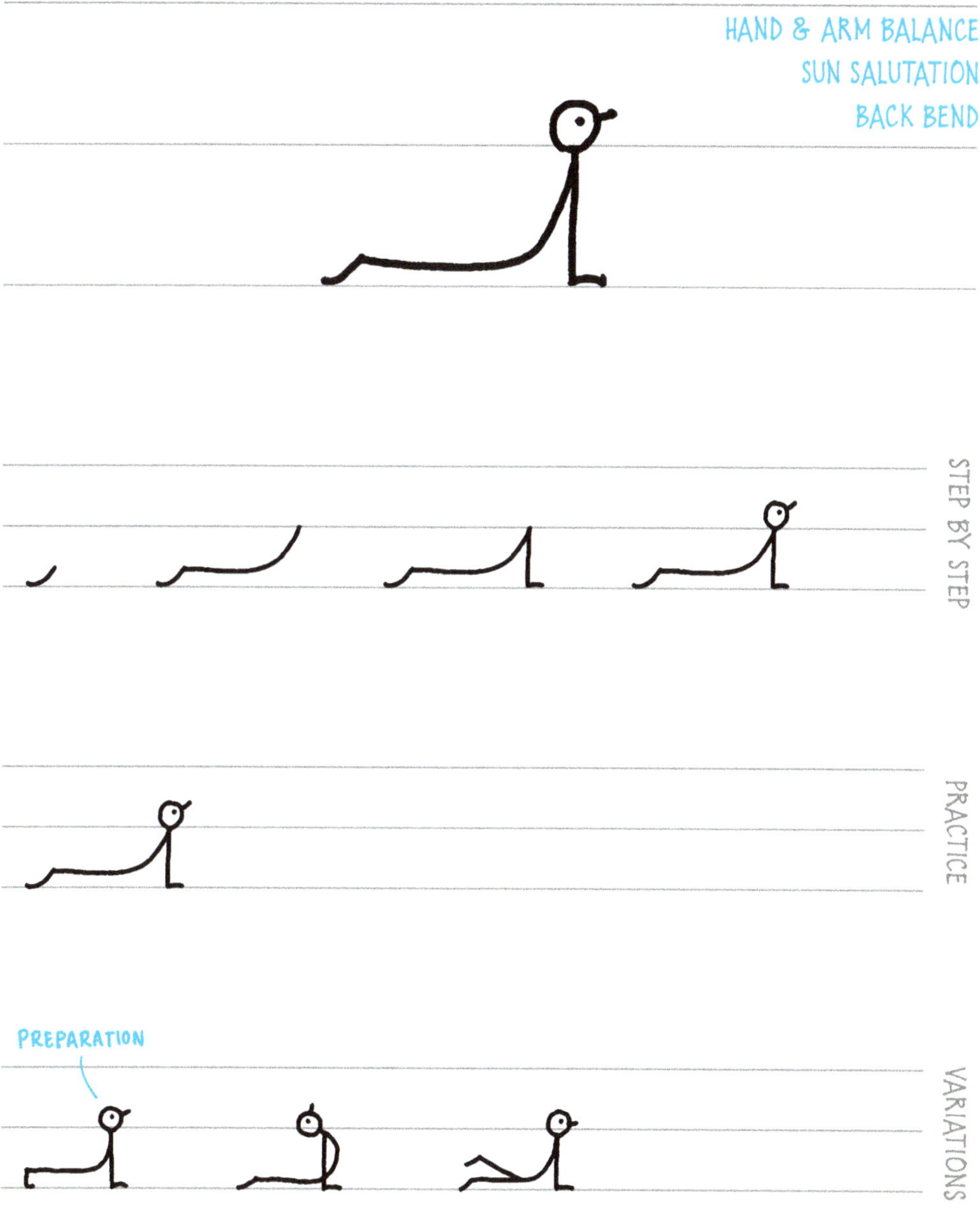

ARDHA PINCHA MAYURASANA

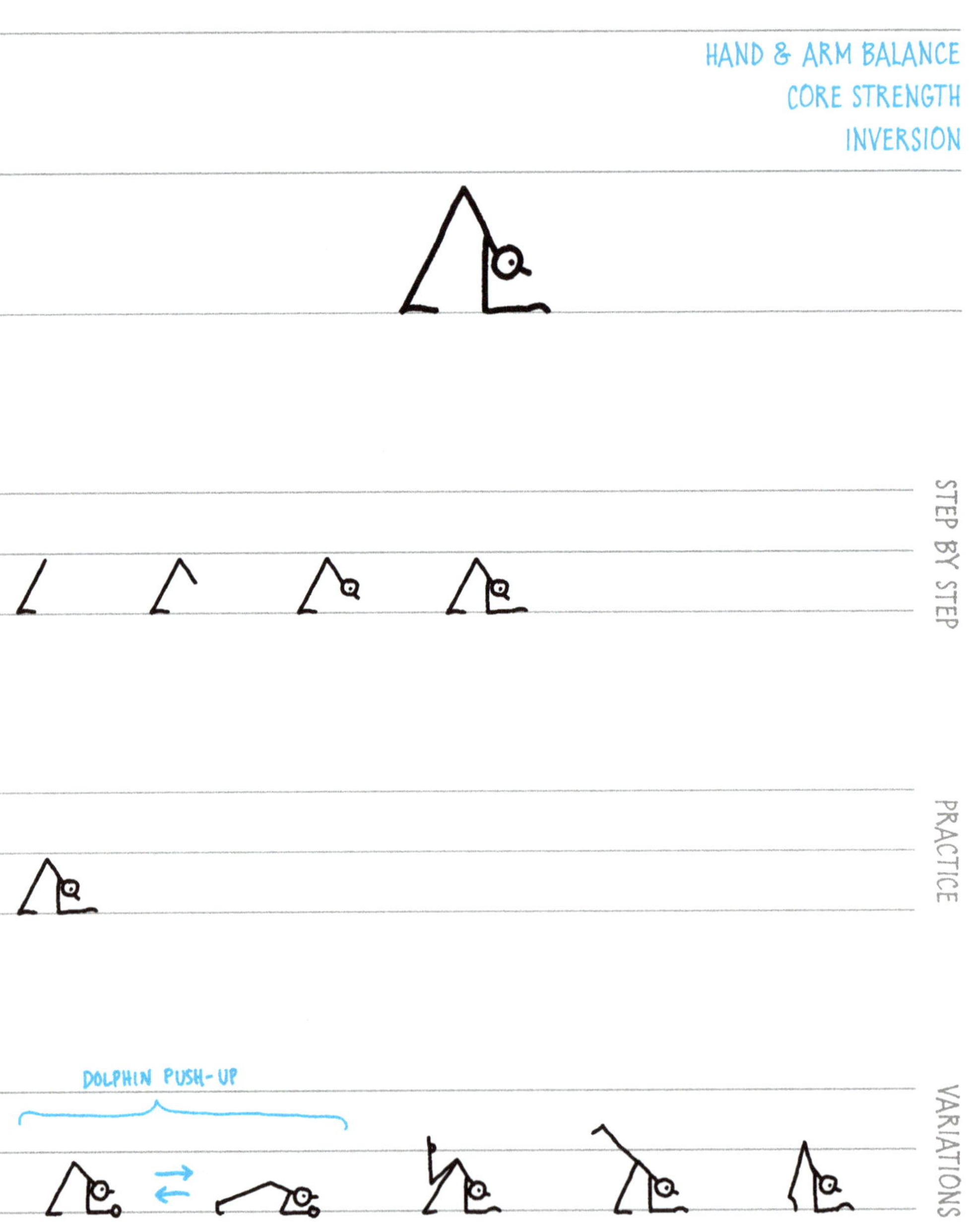

120

PURVOTTASANA

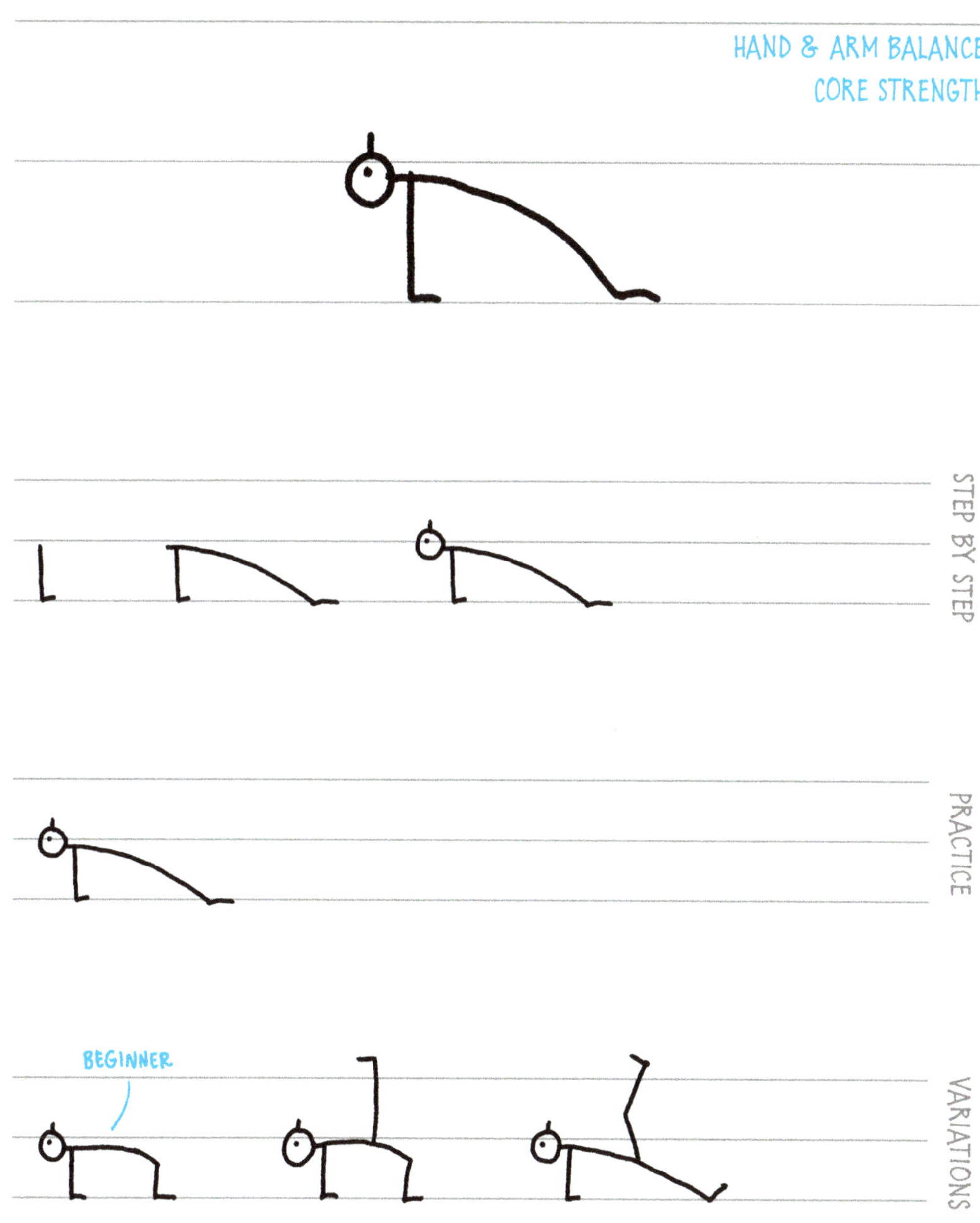

121

BAKASANA
CROW POSE

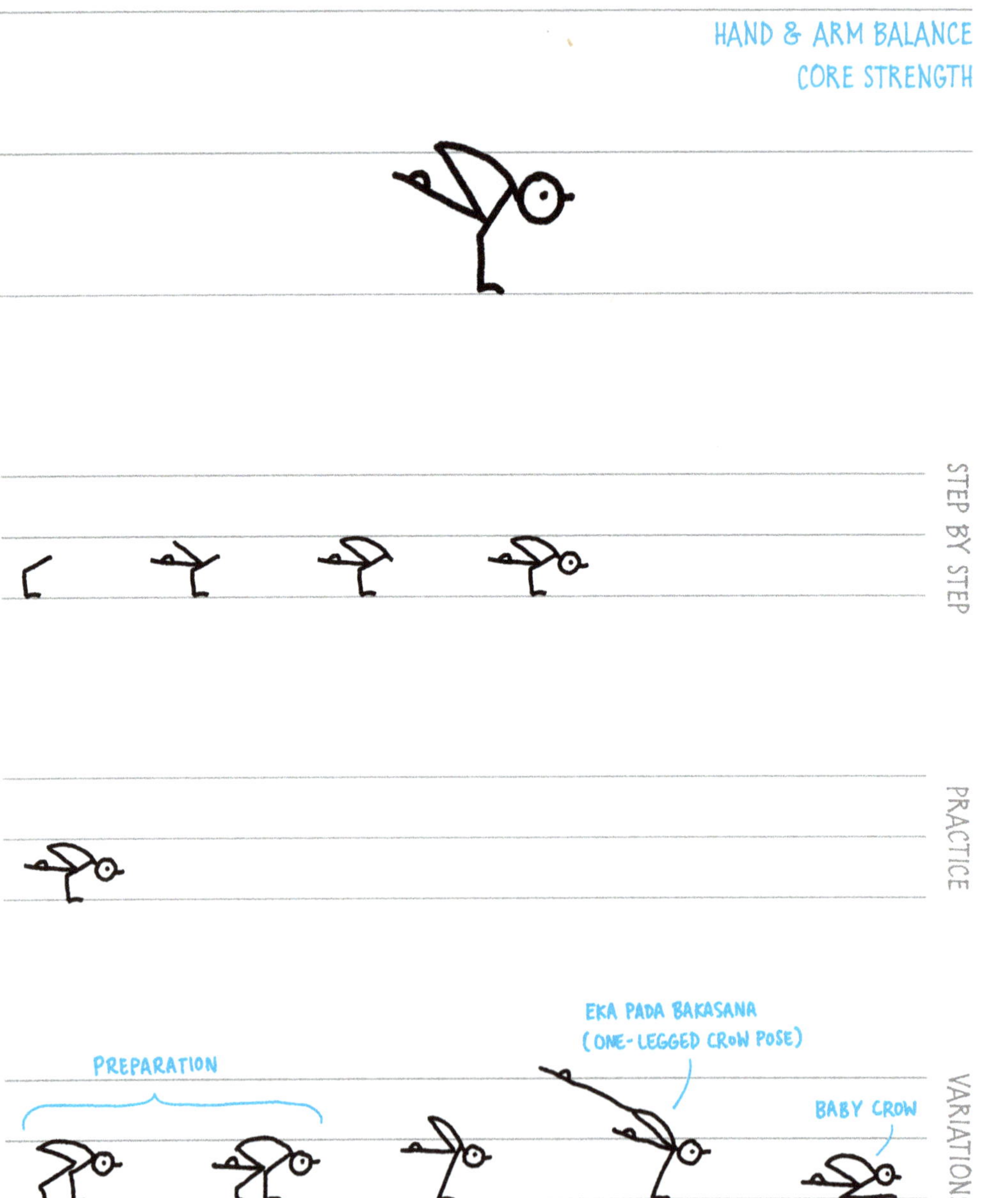

BHUJAPIDASANA

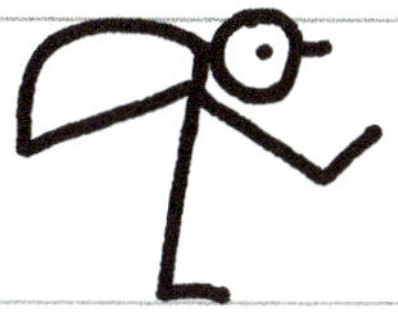

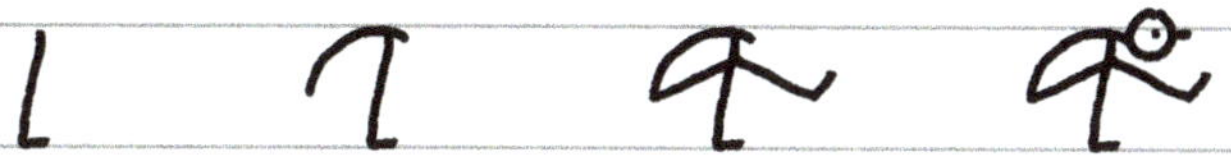

123

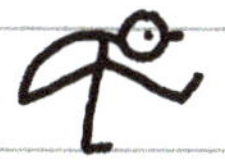

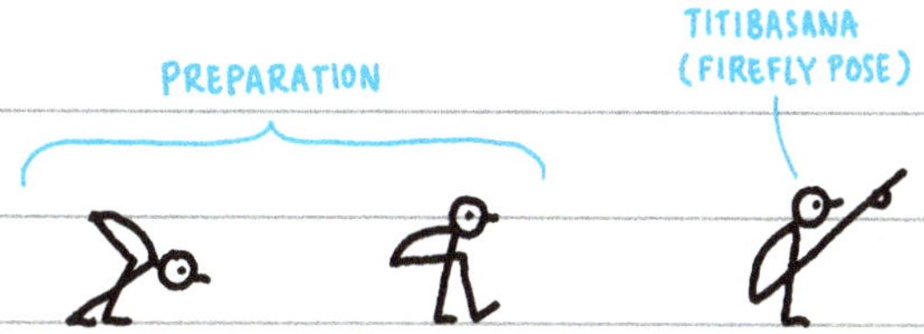

PARSVA BAKASANA

SIDE CROW POSE

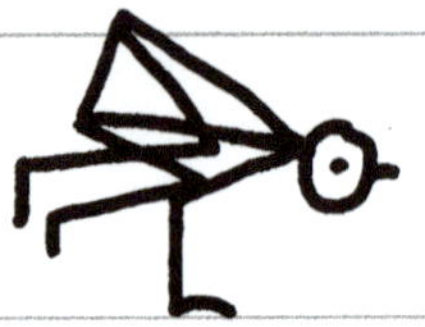

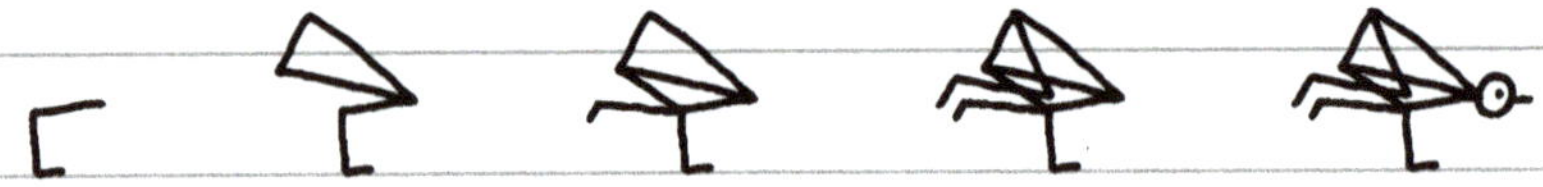

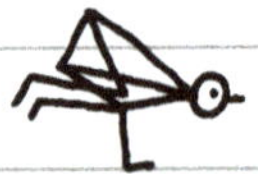

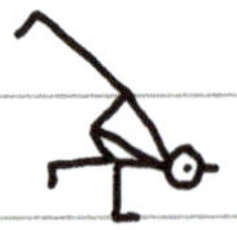

TOLASANA

SCALE POSE

HAND & ARM BALANCE
CORE STRENGTH

STEP BY STEP

PRACTICE

BEGINNER

VARIATIONS

LOLASANA

PENDANT POSE

HAND & ARM BALANCE
CORE STRENGTH

STEP BY STEP

PRACTICE

PREPARATION

BEGINNER

VARIATIONS

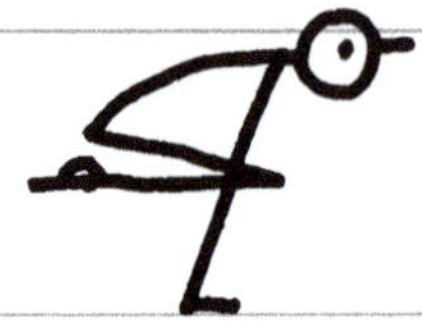

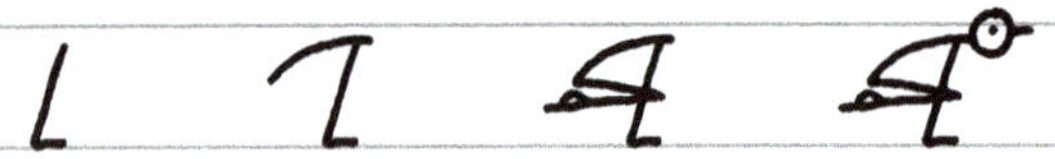

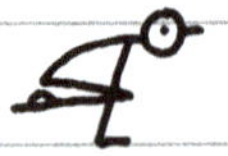

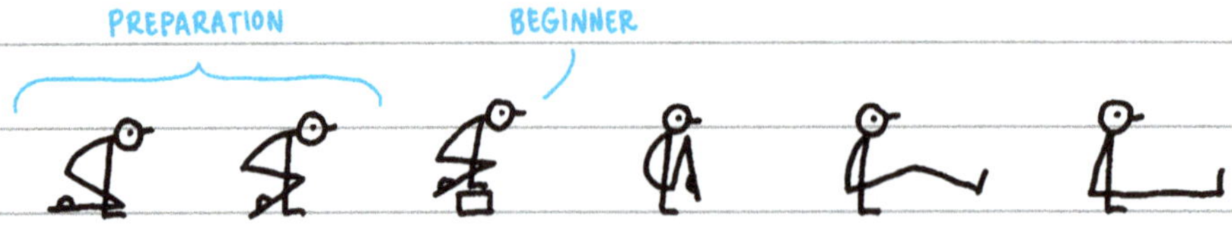

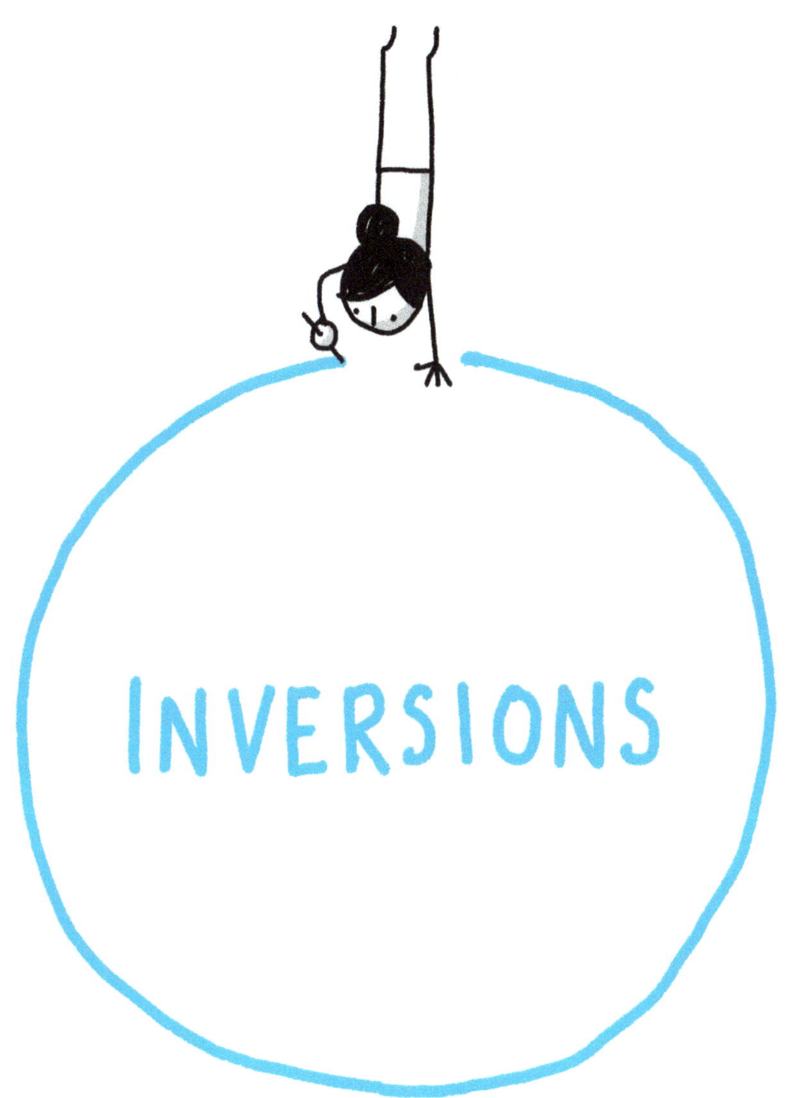

INVERSIONS

SARVANGASANA

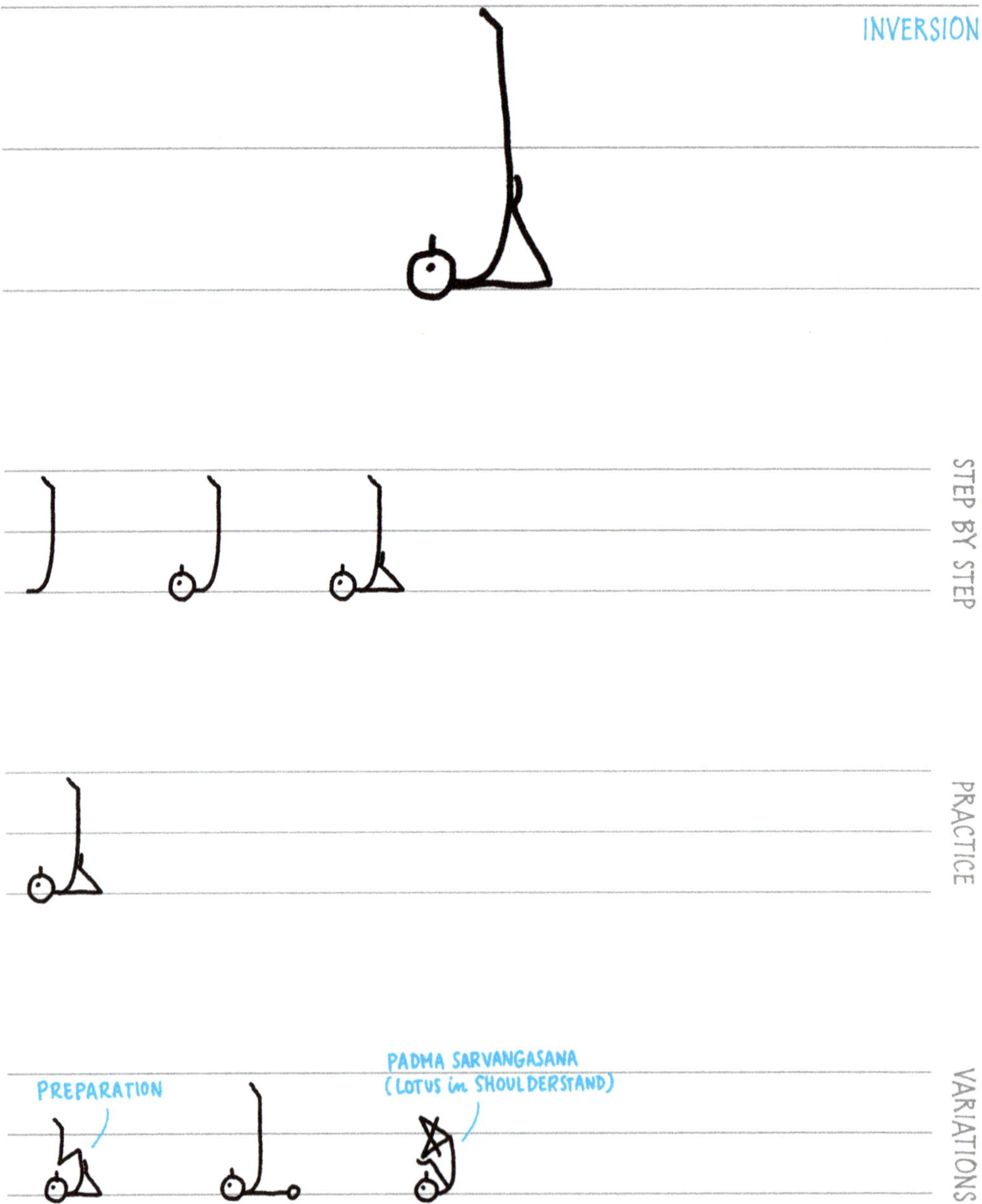

PINCHA MAYURASANA

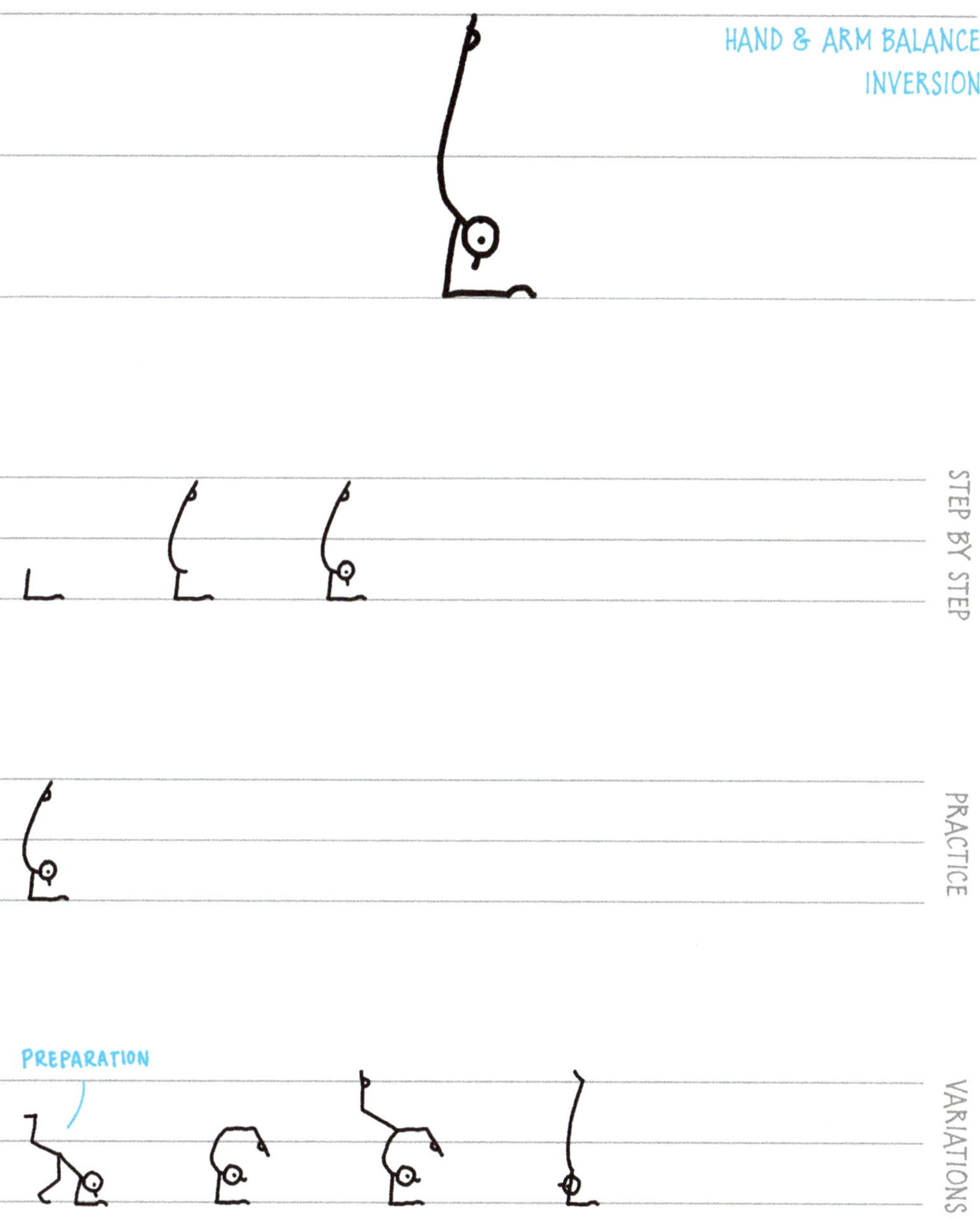

ADHO MUKHA VRKSASANA

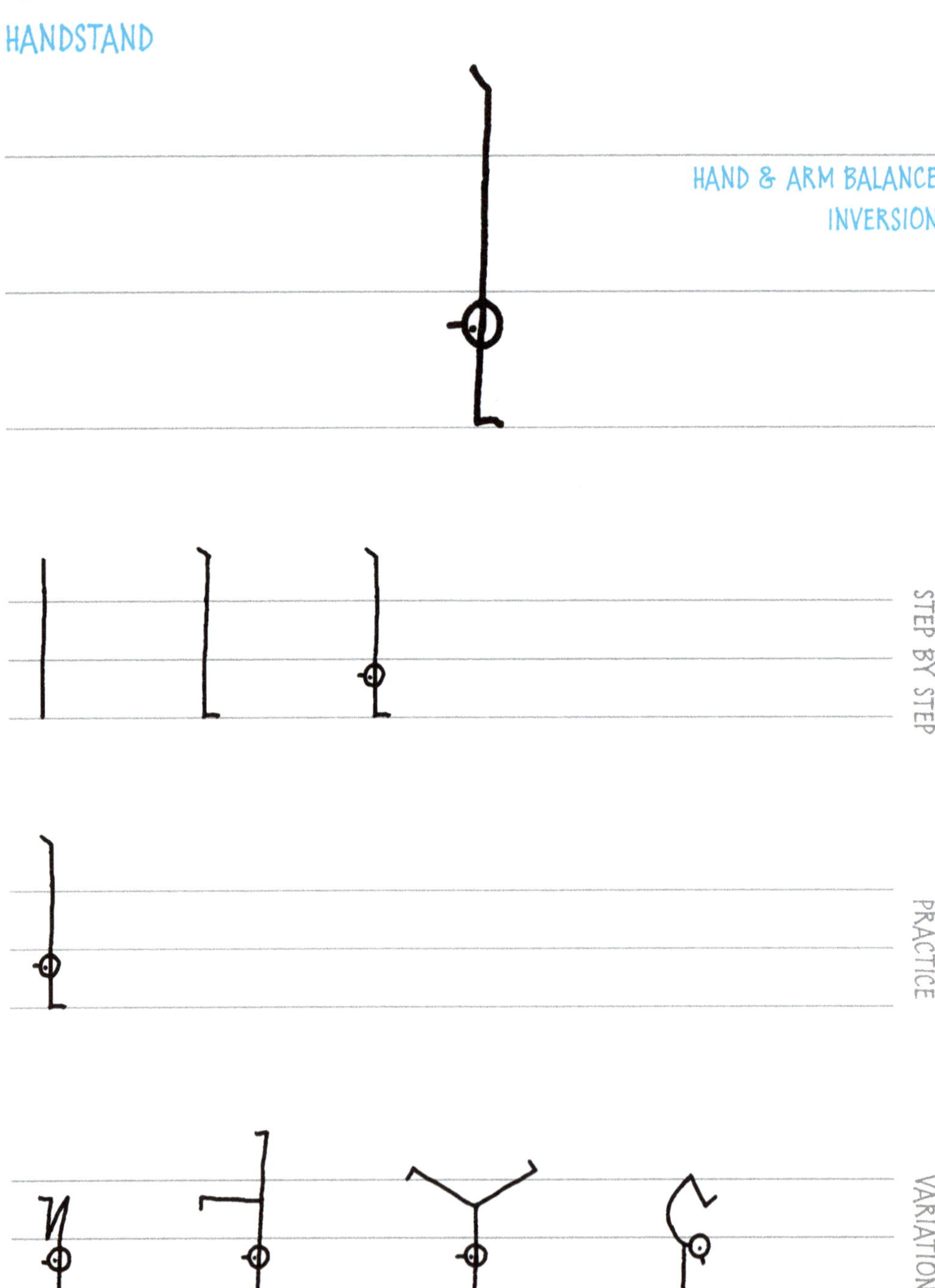

SIRSASANA

HAND & ARM BALANCE
INVERSION
STEP BY STEP
PRACTICE
PREPARATION
MUKTA HASTA SIRSASANA
(TRIPOD HEADSTAND)
VARIATIONS

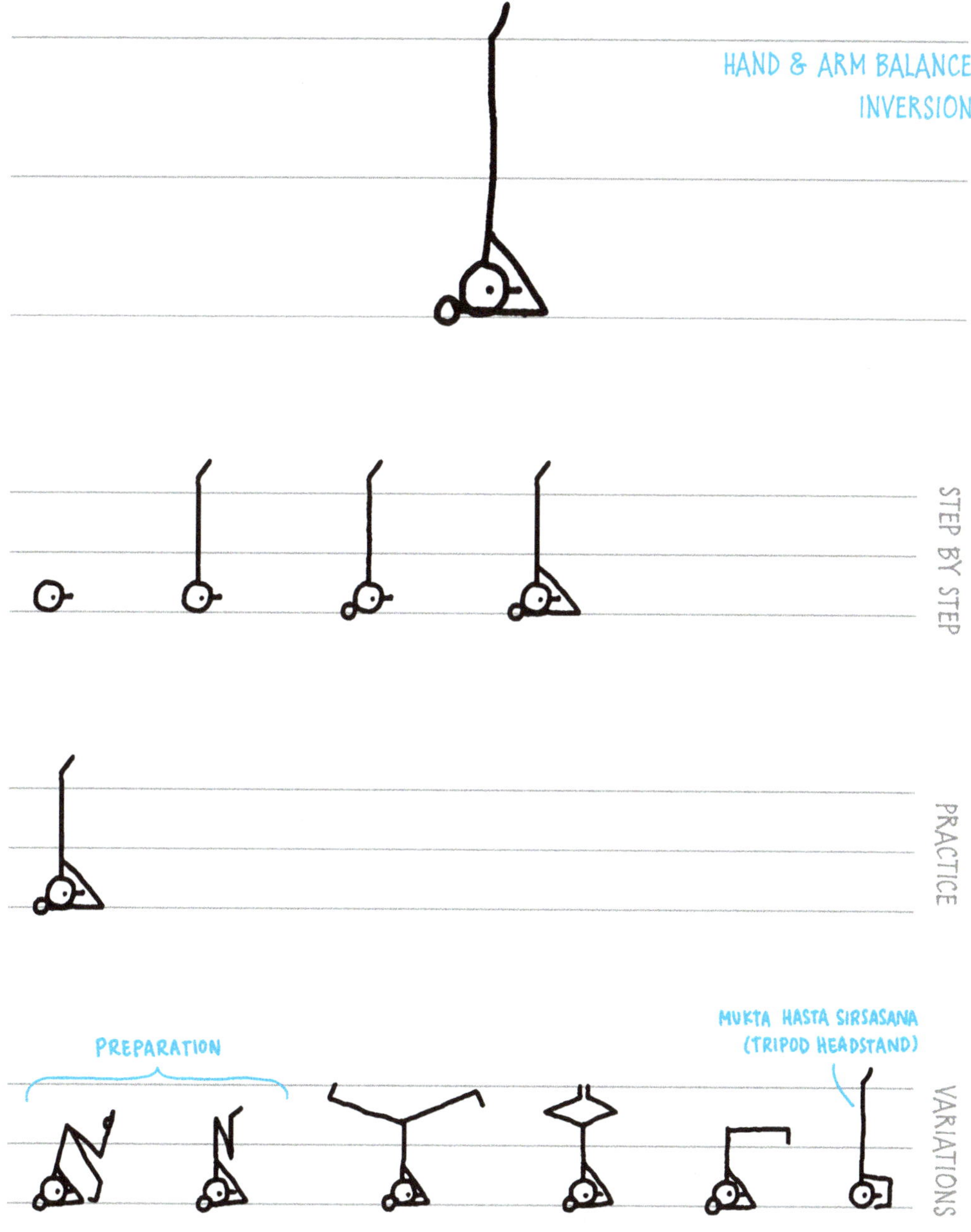

INDEX OF POSTURES – ENGLISH

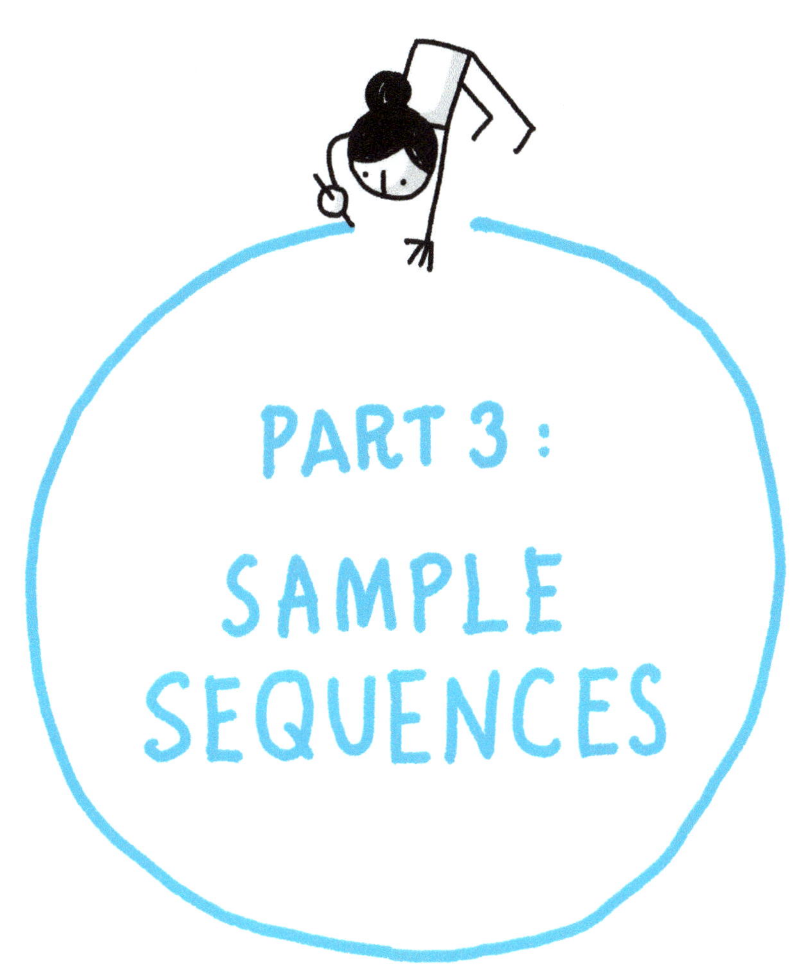

135

SURYA NAMASKAR A

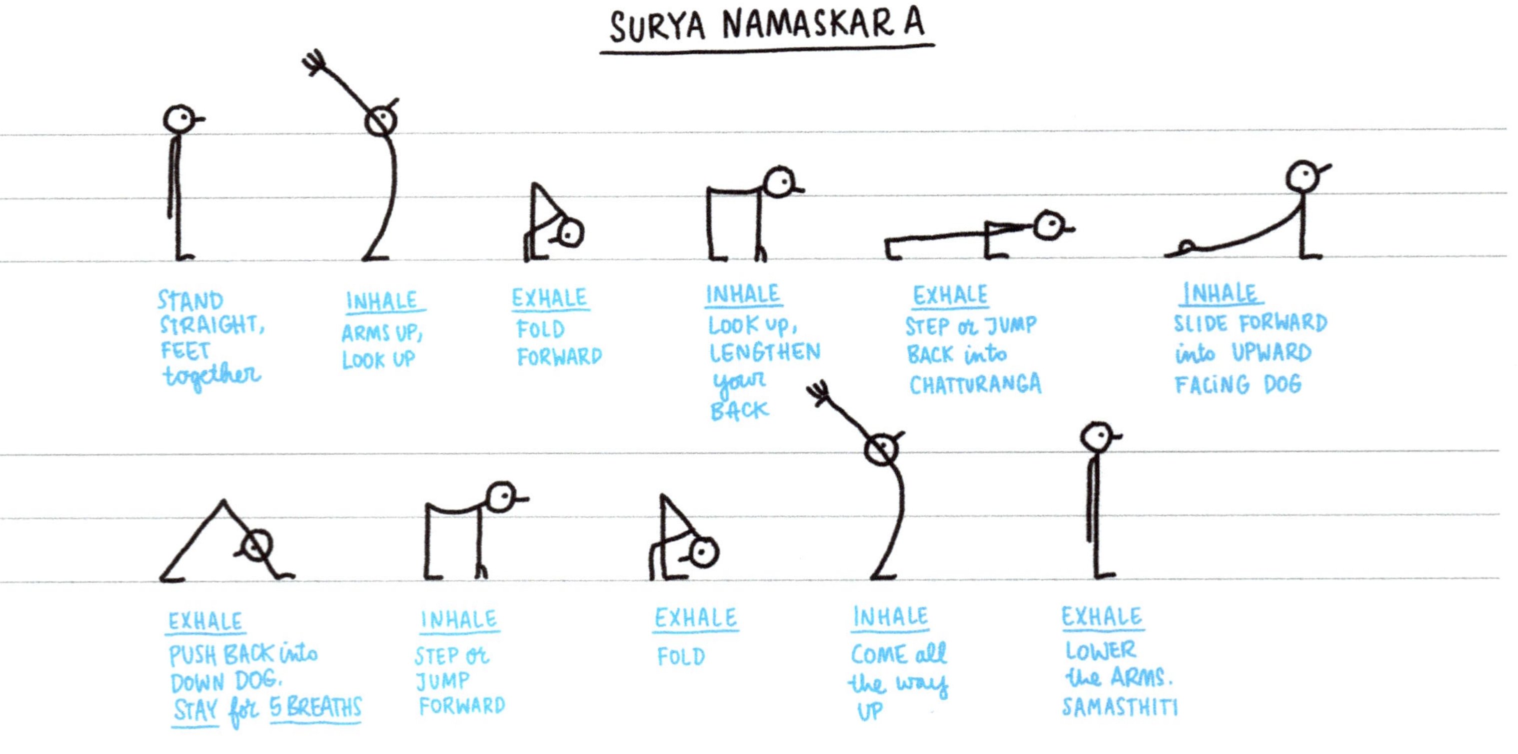

www.yoganotes.net   instagram: @yoga

SURYA NAMASKAR B

STAND STRAIGHT, FEET together

INHALE
BEND your KNEES, RAISE your ARMS

EXHALE
FOLD FORWARD

INHALE
STRAIGHTEN your BACK, LOOK UP

EXHALE
STEP or JUMP BACK into CHATTURANGA

INHALE
SLIDE forward into UP DOG

EXHALE
PUSH BACK into DOWN DOG

INHALE
STEP your RIGHT LEG FORWARD & RAISE your ARMS

EXHALE
STEP BACK into CHATTURANGA

INHALE
PUSH UP into UP DOG

then REPEAT on the LEFT SIDE

EXHALE
PUSH BACK into DOWN DOG. STAY for 5 BREATHS

INHALE
STEP or JUMP FORWARD

EXHALE
FOLD

INHALE
BEND your KNEES, ARMS UP

EXHALE
STAND UP, ARMS DOWN. SAMASTHITI

www.yoganotes.net   instagram: @yoga

SURYA NAMASKAR C

STAND
STRAIGHT,
FEET
together

INHALE &
EXHALE
HANDS to
HEART-CENTER

INHALE
ARMS UP,
LOOK UP

EXHALE
FOLD
FORWARD

INHALE
STEP your RIGHT
LEG BACK, RIGHT
KNEE on the
GROUND

HOLD the BREATH
STEP your LEFT
LEG BACK
into PLANK

EXHALE
LOWER your
KNEES, CHEST &
CHIN onto the
FLOOR

INHALE
SLIDE FORWARD
into COBRA

EXHALE
PUSH BACK
into
DOWN DOG

INHALE
STEP your
LEFT LEG forward,
RIGHT KNEE on
the ground

EXHALE
STEP your
RIGHT LEG
forward to
MEET the LEFT

INHALE
COME all
the way
UP

EXHALE
BRING your
HANDS DOWN
by your SIDES

→ then REPEAT the WHOLE SEQUENCE
on the OTHER SIDE.

www.yoganotes.net   instagram: @yoga

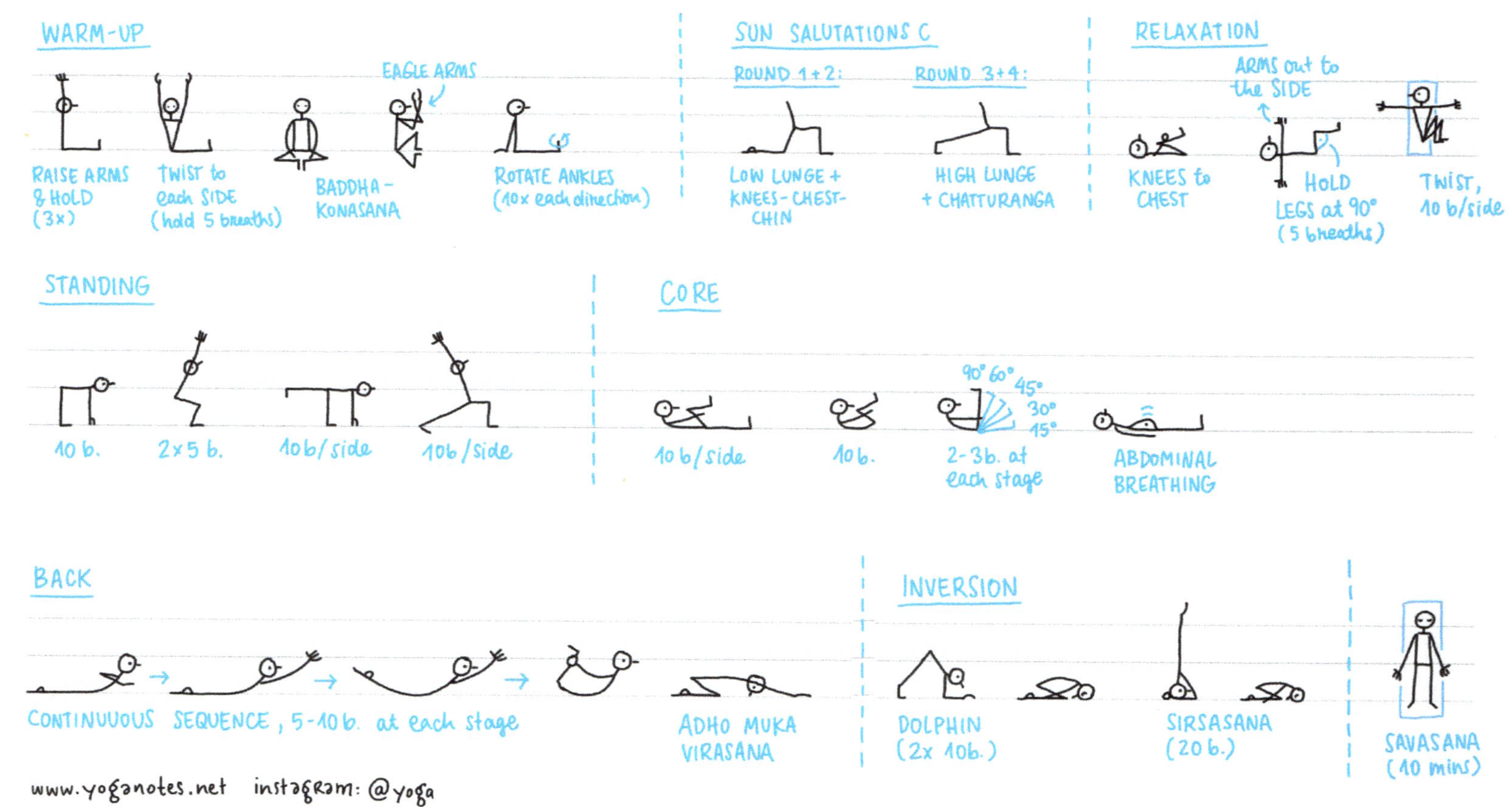

HATHA CLASS - 75 MINUTES

WARM-UP
RAISE ARMS & HOLD (3x)
TWIST to each SIDE (hold 5 breaths)
EAGLE ARMS
BADDHA-KONASANA
ROTATE ANKLES (10x each direction)

SUN SALUTATIONS C
ROUND 1+2:
LOW LUNGE + KNEES-CHEST-CHIN
ROUND 3+4:
HIGH LUNGE + CHATTURANGA

RELAXATION
KNEES to CHEST
ARMS out to the SIDE
HOLD LEGS at 90° (5 breaths)
TWIST, 10 b/side

STANDING
10 b.
2x5 b.
10 b/side
10 b/side

CORE
10 b/side
10 b.
90° 60° 45° 30° 15°
2-3 b. at each stage
ABDOMINAL BREATHING

BACK
CONTINUUOUS SEQUENCE, 5-10 b. at each stage
ADHO MUKA VIRASANA

INVERSION
DOLPHIN (2x 10 b.)
SIRSASANA (20 b.)

SAVASANA (10 mins)

www.yoganotes.net   instagram: @yoga

ABOUT EVA-LOTTA LAMM

Eva-Lotta is a designer, illustrator and visual thinker. After studying design in Germany, she lived in Paris and London for 10 years, working as a User Experience designer for companies like Yahoo, Skype and Google.

She is also known for taking sketchnotes — a hand drawn form of visual notes that combine words and images into rich visual summaries — at design conferences around the globe. She published her sketchnotes in several books.

Eva-Lotta is a sought after expert and speaker on the topic of sketching and visual thinking. She regularly teaches sketching workshops, helping people from all kinds of professions to use the power of visual thinking to develop and express their ideas.

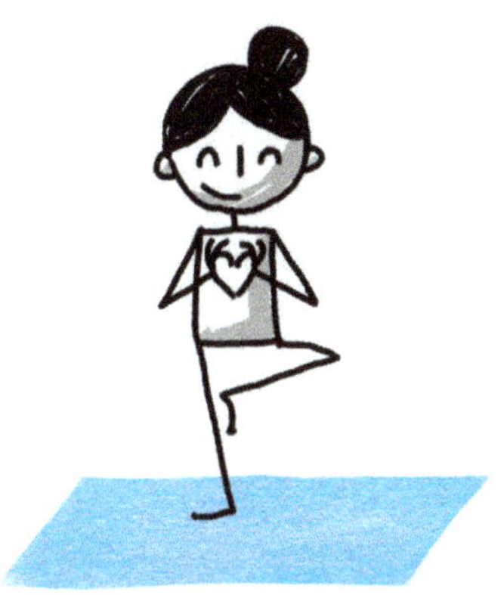

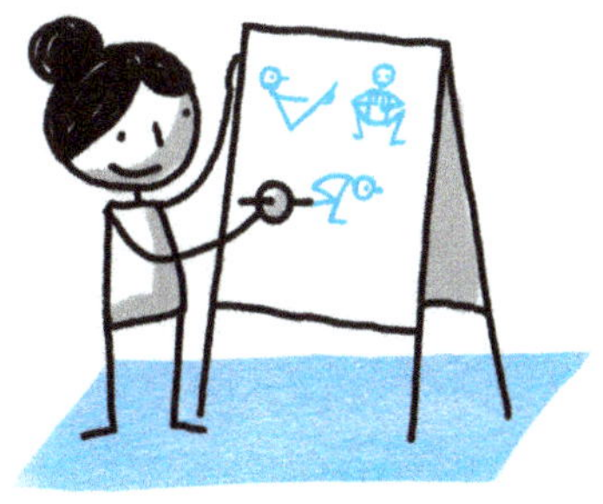

Her yoga journey began in 2013 when she got introduced to Shivananda Yoga in London. After trying out various styles and classes, she found her teacher Surinder Singh on a trip to India in Rishikesh in 2014. With him, she studied classic Hatha Yoga. She returned in 2016 to complete a teacher training course and practice in the shala for several months. Her visual notes from the course are available as a book.

After being a (semi-)nomad for over 2 years — travelling the world, studying yoga and improvisation and doing freelance work — she now lives in Berlin, working as an independent designer, teacher and author.

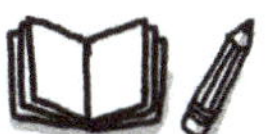

LEARN MORE ABOUT
EVA-LOTTA'S
WORK & BOOKS

www.evalotta.net
www.evalotta.shop

FOLLOW
EVA-LOTTA
ON SOCIAL MEDIA

Instagram: @evalottchen
Twitter: @evalottchen
Facebook: Eva-Lotta Lamm

BECOME PART OF
THE #YOGANOTES
COMMUNITY

Instagram: @yoga.notes
Facebook: sketchyoganotes
Web: www.yoganotes.net

MORE BOOKS AND PRODUCTS BY EVA-LOTTA

I love creating things that help people learn, inspire them to express themselves
or just bring a smile to their face. You can find them all at **www.evalotta.shop**

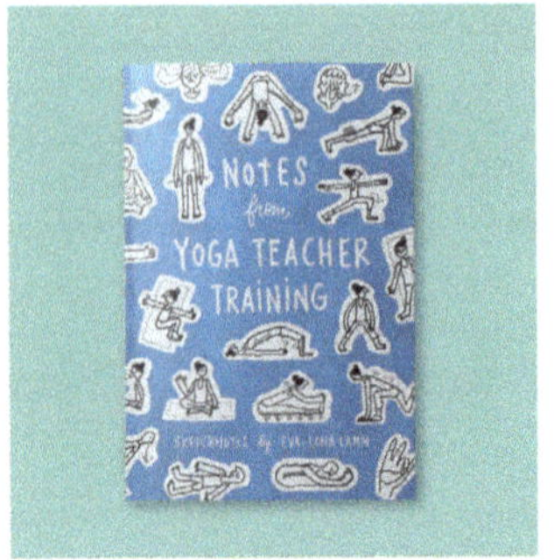

←
Notes from Yoga Teacher Training
Sketchnotes from my 200-hour Hatha Yoga TTC in Rishikesh, India.

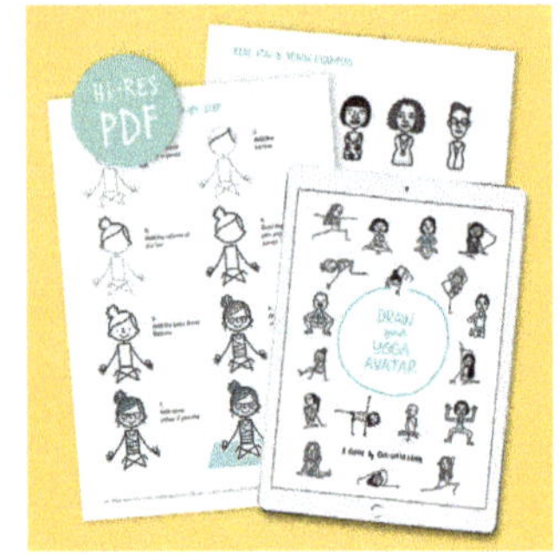

↑
Draw your Yoga-Avatar
Learn to draw friendly yoga avatars for yourself and all your yoga friends.

→
Illustrated Sanskrit Words
A set of illustrated charts presenting 77 key Sanskrit words to understand yoga asana names.

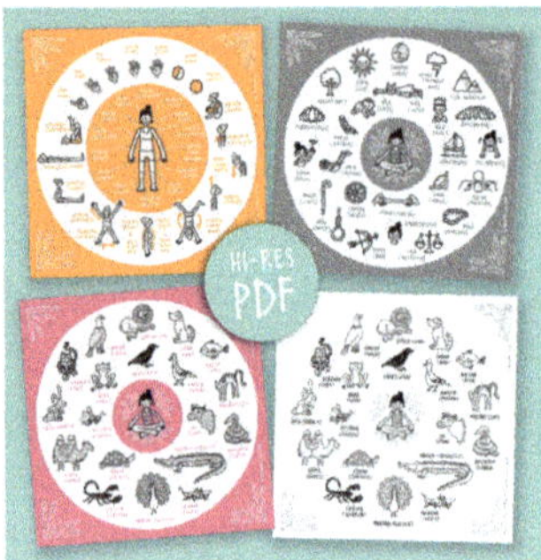

Yoganotes Online Workshop
If you prefer learning by video instructions, there is also an online workshop teaching you the basics of sketching simple but clear yoga stick figures.
↓

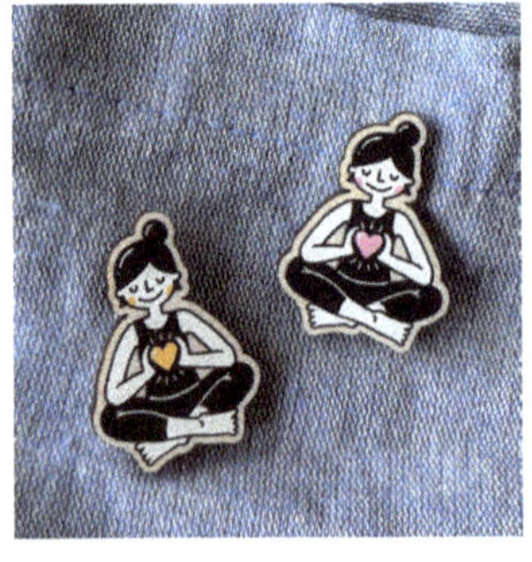

↑
Wooden Yogini Pins
The perfect little accessory for passionate yogi/nis, made from responsibly sourced birch wood.

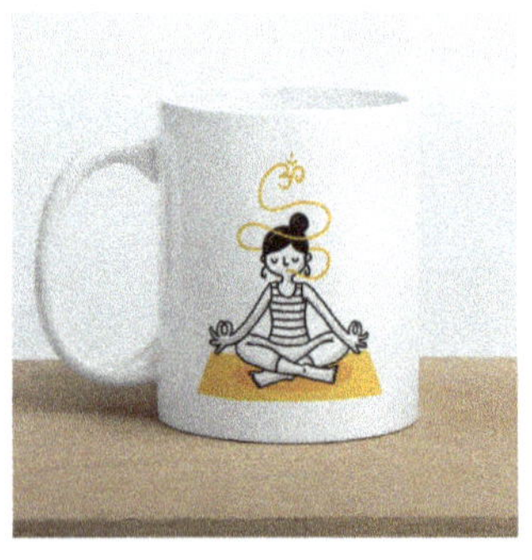

↑
Yogini mugs
Beautiful ceramic mugs featuring yoginis in different poses.

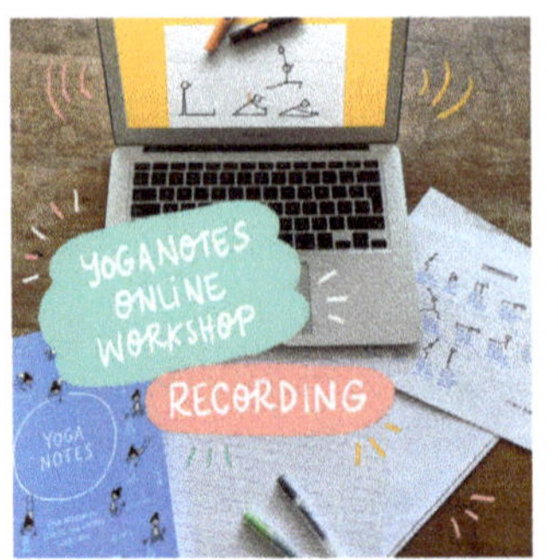

www.evalotta.shop

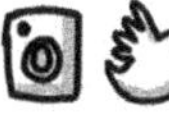

@evalottchen

Berlin · 2020